Clinical Oral Medicine

CLINICAL ORAL MEDICINE

J. J. GAYFORD

MB BS, BDS, MRC Psych, FDS RCS (Eng), MRCS, LRCP, AKC
Consultant Psychiatrist
Previously, Lecturer in Oral Medicine,
Institute of Dental Surgery, London

and

R. HASKELL

MB BS, BDS, MRCP, FDS RCS(Eng)
Consultant Oral Surgeon,
Guy's Hospital, London

With a Foreword by
SIR ROBERT BRADLAW
CBE, FRCS, FDS RCS
Honorary Professor of Oral Pathology,
Royal College of Surgeons of England;
Emeritus Professor of Oral Medicine,
University of London

Second edition
Revised by R. HASKELL

BRISTOL
JOHN WRIGHT & SONS LTD
1979

First edition, 1971
(Published by Staples Press)
Second edition, 1979

CIP Data

Gayford, Jasper John
  Clinical oral medicine.—2nd ed.
  1. Mouth—Diseases
  2. Face—Diseases
  I. Title   II. Haskell, Richard
  617'.52   RC815

ISBN 0 7236 0512 2

Text set in 11/12 pt Photon Times, printed and bound
in Great Britain at The Pitman Press, Bath

Preface

Since the appearance of the first edition there have been developments of some significance in the understanding and management of oral ulceration and temporomandibular joint dysfunction which have necessitated rewriting those sections. A new chapter on the tongue has been added and there has been updating and revision of most chapters.

At a more personal level Dr Gayford has taken up a career in psychiatry so the revisions for this edition have been left to me. I would like to record my thanks to Professor R. A. Cawson, Dr W. H. Binnie and Dr M. Wilton for discussions over the past few years which have illuminated my understanding of many topics, which I hope is reflected in the text.

There are moves afoot to introduce a separate examination in Oral Medicine and Pathology in London University BDS finals. This I deplore since dental surgery (or stomatology) is neither sufficiently large nor complex to require this interminable subdivision. It is, however, a reflection of the growing recognition of oral medicine in undergraduate education—a beneficial change.

1979

R.H.

Errata
p. 132, line 10. *For* Stomatisis *read* Stomatitis.
pp. 266, 267. The illustrations for *Figs.* 11 and 12 should be transposed.

Contents

List of Plates

(*Following* p. 276)

Foreword

It is a relatively short time since the first chair in Oral Medicine was established in a British University. The increase of knowledge both in basic medical science and its clinical application has unavoidably encouraged specialisation; this makes it essential that the busy clinician should have access to these developments in a convenient form so that he can assess their significance in his own field.

The second edition of this deservedly successful textbook will enable him to do this. Clinical experience has enabled the authors to give appropriate emphasis to what is important and to refer only briefly to conditions which are seen infrequently. Some measure of condensation has been unavoidable if a proper balance was to be ensured. There is an excellent bibliography at the end of each chapter.

Good wine needs no bush but this is undoubtedly the best work of its kind that I have read. I can recommend it to students for whom it will provide a sound foundation and to clinicians as a comprehensive survey and a most useful source of reference.

Introduction

To both doctors and dentists alike, the mouth represents an important part of the body which suffers diseases peculiar to it and is also frequently involved in many systemic disorders. Oral medicine may be defined as the diagnosis and treatment of 'medical' conditions of the mouth and associated structures. However, the practice of oral medicine, as defined above, is divided between the medical and dental professions, sometimes to the detriment of the patient. No plea is being made for the recognition of oral medicine as a separate speciality spanning medicine and dentistry, yet there is a place for practitioners with a sound knowledge of the subject. For teaching purposes and research, specialization in particular subjects, including oral medicine, is required.

The mouth and face cannot be divorced from the patient as a whole and one of the fascinations of oral medicine is that it may lead the clinician into all the branches of medicine and dentistry. Often it is difficult to know when to call a halt but any clinician must have the humility to refer a case, however interesting, to a colleague better equipped to continue the patient's treatment. This is easier if colleagues have an understanding of each others' speciality, so that a study of oral medicine should lead to better cooperation between medical and dental practitioners.

This book is hopefully directed to a wide audience; firstly to medical and dental practitioners. We also hope that specialists in medicine, surgery and dentistry will feel richer for an understanding of oral medicine, especially as they are so often called upon to practise this subject — generally unaware that they have departed from their own sphere of activity. Secondly, the needs of postgraduate dental students have been considered since experience of teaching them has emphasized the need for a text to cover their requirements. Doctors are asked to bear with thumbnail sketches of systemic disorders which are intended for dental surgeons whose indulgence is likewise craved while dental conditions are described for medical readers.

Very little pathology has been included which in no way reflects our estimation of that subject but rather the fact that there are several excellent texts of oral pathology, so we have confined ourselves to clinical features. For the same reason, purely dental diseases have been largely ignored.

Acknowledgements

We wish to thank Professor Sir Robert V. Bradlaw, CBE, MDS, FRCS, late Dean of the Institute of Dental Surgery and Director of the Eastman Dental Hospital, for allowing us to reproduce Plates 21, 23, 29, 30 and 31, and for information related to cases under his care.

Dr W. Gooddy, MD, FRCP, consultant neurologist to the National Hospital, Queen's Square and University College Hospital, London, kindly read the chapters related to neurology and offered helpful advice. We would also like to thank all our colleagues, medical and dental, for helpful discussion and criticism. Illustrations have been kindly prepared by the Photographic Department of the Eastman Dental Hospital and some by a colleague, Dr Philip Merdin, MB, CHB.

Finally, we record our deep indebtedness to the secretaries who have prepared the manuscript, in particular Mrs B. Rayiru and Miss N. Valère.

January 1971   J. J. G.   R. H.

Chapter 1

Oral Ulceration

Introduction. In this chapter will be considered the major causes of oral ulceration (excluding neoplastic disease) which are not preceded by vesiculobullous lesions.

They will be considered under the following main headings:

1. Recurrent aphthous ulceration.
2. Behçet's syndrome.
3. Reiter's syndrome.
   (digression) Human lymphatic antigen system and oral ulceration.
4. Necrotizing sialometaplasia.
5. Agranulocytosis and neutropenia.

Recurrent Aphthous Ulceration

Aphthous ulcers are persistently recurrent, painful ulcers of the oral mucosa, of unknown aetiology. It seems probable that presently grouped together are a heterogenous collection of clinical entities.

Synonyms

There is much confusion caused by the large number of names that have been used to describe this condition: such terms as aphthous stomatitis, canker sore, dyspeptic ulcers, habitual ulcers, mucosal ulcers, Mikulicz's ulcers, ulcer necroticum mucosae oris and ulcers neuroticum mucosae oris are to be seen in the literature.

Variants of aphthous ulcers

Not all aphthous ulcers have the same clinical features. There is considerable variation in size, depth and length of persistence. Where the ulcers are large, penetrating into the deeper tissues with associated submandibular lymphadenopathy, the term 'major aphthae' may be used, or

1

alternatively, 'periadenitis mucosa necrotica recurrens'. This type of ulcer lasts much longer and heals with a scar.

Patients presenting with multiple small ulcers the size of a pinhead have been described under the term 'herpetiform aphthous ulcers'. Not all agree that this type of ulcer should be regarded as a variant of aphthous ulcer but should be regarded as a viral-induced ulcer. Attractive though this view may be, there is no proof to substantiate it.

Incidence

This varies according to the section of the population sampled. No figures less than 10 per cent have been quoted for any population survey. Of patients who are attending hospital outpatient departments for any condition, the incidence is 20 per cent and in selected groups figures as high as 60 per cent have been recorded. Females are more commonly affected than males, probably in the ratio 3:2. Ulcers may start in childhood, but do so more usually in the teenager. In most cases they become less frequent as the patient enters the fourth decade and may fade in the fifth and sixth decades of life. Women seem to persist with their ulcers longer than men and may start at an earlier age.

Aetiology and pathogenesis

As stated above, the aetiology is unknown. Many interesting hypotheses have been put forward with their associated groups of supporters, each is held enthusiastically for a time and then fades to be replaced by a new theory which reflects current research.

It is proposed to mention briefly some of the aetiological factors that have been cited.

1. *Heredity:* About 50 per cent of patients have a history of one parent having aphthous ulcers; it is much rarer for both parents to have the condition. Siblings are not always affected and it would be very rare indeed to find a large family suffering in this way. Sircus was of the opinion that where two parents were involved there could be anticipation in the age of occurrence with some of their children.

2. *Trauma:* This is supported by the clinical observation that some patients develop a crop of ulcers following minor trauma to the oral mucosa. Commonly this follows routine dental treatment, where even the presence of a cotton-wool roll in the mouth or the injection of a local

anaesthetic may produce ulceration. Many cases occur with no history of previous trauma.

3. *Infection:* This may be divided into (a) bacterial and (b) viral.

  a. Bacterial: the recent isolation of transitional L-form bacteria from aphthous ulcers has revived this idea. Transitional L-form bacteria may be classified as mycoplasma but have many features in common with streptococci. Hopeful though this theory may have seemed to some workers, the finding of these organisms is not persistent, nor is their presence confined to aphthous ulcers. Koch's postulates have in no way been demonstrated.

  b. Viral: this theory was more in vogue before the appropriate techniques were available for the investigation of viruses. Although it has not been possible constantly to isolate any virus, much work has been done assuming that *Herpes simplex* is the causative agent. The outcome of this has been slightly surprising in that patients with recurrent aphthous ulceration have been shown to have a lower incidence of *Herpes simplex* antibodies than the control sample of subjects with no history of aphthous ulceration. Nevertheless, claims have been made for the isolation of *Herpes simplex* antibodies in recurrent herpetiform ulceration and even giant cells have been found. There is a great deal more evidence and constant results needed before these theories can be accepted.

4. *Association with gastrointestinal disturbances:* About 30 per cent of patients with aphthous ulcers have an associated history of dyspepsia, but the incidence of proven peptic ulceration is no higher than in the general public. Aphthous ulcers are extremely frequent in patients with ulcerative colitis. Oral ulceration of 'aphthous' type is not uncommon in coeliac disease and a prominent and early feature of tropical sprue.

  An extremely interesting observation was reported in 1976 by Ferguson et al. that of 33 patients with severe recurrent oral ulceration 8 had jejunal mucosal biopsy specimens with typical histological features of coeliac disease (none of these patients had evidence of malabsorption or clinical features of coeliac disease). Furthermore, treatment with a gluten-free diet produced considerable improvement in the oral ulceration. Unfortunately these observations have not been confirmed (Cawson and Lehner, personal communication).

  Tropical sprue is a malabsorption syndrome of unknown aetiology occurring in Asia and the Caribbean, often with acute enteritic onset, associated with folate deficiency and malabsorption of vitamin B_{12},

D-xylose, fat and nutrients. It may be considerably helped by folic acid but far better results occur if that is supplemented by broad-spectrum antibiotics, while vitamin B_{12} is also required if tissue stores are lowered by chronic disease. The aetiology remains unknown. The oral ulceration accompanying sprue may well be associated with the folate and vitamin B_{12} deficiency (*see below*), due to malabsorption or be related in an entirely different way to the aetiological agent. By all accounts extensive oral ulceration clinically similar to aphthous ulceration is a prominent feature.

5. *Association with atopy:* Twenty per cent of patients with aphthous ulcers have a history of asthma, eczema or hay fever.

6. *Hormonal influence:* In women a crop of aphthous ulcers is often noted premenstrually and many more women have a cyclic occurrence of ulcers. Other observers have reported that the incidence of aphthous ulceration falls during pregnancy. Bishop et al. claim that there is a group of female patients in whom there would appear to be an endocrine factor. Many of these patients suffered from associated dysmenorrhoea.

7. *Emotional factors:* Fifty per cent of females and 33 per cent of males show a clear emotional factor which may precipitate crops of ulcers. The high incidence found in some groups of young girls preparing for examinations is a clear pointer. Other factors which have already been cited could be indirectly due to emotional factors, e.g. association with dyspepsia and premenstrual tension. Many other patients relate crops of ulcers to periods of stress in their professional or domestic life. Just over 30 per cent of patients in one series investigated showed established features of neuroses. Most commonly this was a mild anxiety state, but obsessional features were not unusual. Depressive features are seen on rare occasions.

8. *The question of auto-immunity:* It is currently very fashionable to claim that diseases of previously unknown aetiology are due to auto-immunity. Aphthous ulceration is no exception to this. Lehner makes a strong case for auto-immunity being an aetiological factor, he claims that in a high proportion of patients with recurrent aphthous ulceration it is possible to demonstrate antibodies to fetal oral mucosa by haemagglutination, complement-fixation and precipitation techniques. Immunofluorescent histochemical techniques were used to show cell-bound antibodies in the tissue surrounding aphthous ulcers. He admits

that this fulfils only two of Witebsky's criteria for auto-immunity, but there are very few conditions that are accepted as auto-immune disease which fulfil all these criteria.

Nevertheless, it is possible to demonstrate auto-antibodies in many cases where there is chronic tissue destruction. The antibodies are caused by the tissue damage and are not the cause of the lesion.

Immediately before ulceration occurs there is an accumulation of lymphocytes which *may* indicate that these cells are of prime significance in causing destruction of the epithelium. Why the lymphocytes accumulate is not clear—either in response to altered epithelium or extrinsic antigenic assault.

Dolby has shown that *in vitro* oral epithelium in tissue culture may be damaged by lymphocytes from patients with aphthous ulceration and that this cytopathogenic action is inhibited by antilymphocytic serum. Similar damage to epithelial cells could not be produced by serum containing antimucosal antibodies from aphthous ulcer patients and the lymphocytic action was not enhanced by serum.

Thus lymphocytes may play a role in the pathogenesis of aphthous ulcers.

9. *Haematological factors:* Wray et al. have shown that investigation to exclude iron, vitamin-B_{12} and folate deficiency is essential since in many cases such deficiency may be associated with aphthous ulceration. In practice it is sufficient to carry out haemoglobin and red cell estimations (including film) to exclude macrocytic anaemia but a serum iron is essential as it is very common to find recurrent 'aphthous' ulceration associated with iron deficiency without anaemia (sideropenia). It is also true, however, that many people with iron deficiency, even if anaemic, do not develop recurrent oral ulceration. Equally anaemia (or iron deficiency) may predispose to candidal infection and to *erosive* episodes in lichen planus.

Important figures from the Glasgow work include the following (130 patients):

   a. 17·7 per cent of patients had Fe^{++} folate or vitamin-B_{12} deficiency as compared with 8·5 per cent of controls.

   b. Of 15 iron-deficient patients only 4 were anaemic.

   c. Five patients were shown to have gluten-sensitive enteropathy of whom 4 had folate-deficiency anaemia.

   d. Five patients were vitamin-B_{12} deficient of whom 3 had anaemia while 2 had no evidence of the deficiency in the peripheral blood.

All patients responded beneficially to treatment of the deficiency —two-thirds of them showing complete remission of oral ulceration.

This work has been confirmed but Lehner has interpreted the findings as indicating a progressive iron deficiency *resulting* from recurrent aphthous ulceration.

Clinical features

The clinical picture of minor aphthous ulcers will be described separately from the two variants, major and herpetiform aphthous ulcers, although they may be seen in the same patient. All occur at the same sites in the mouth, i.e. on the non-keratinized mucosa. On rare occasions aphthous ulcers may be seen on the dorsum of the tongue when they appear as the small type of lesion.

Minor Aphthous ulcers: The patient is aware of pain or soreness in an area of the mouth. He may notice that the mucosa is nodular. If the lateral margin of the tongue is involved, there may be hyperaesthesia. At this stage the only physical sign is an area of erythematous mucous membrane. Within 24 hours the mucous membrane breaks down to form a small ulcer which increases in size for the next few days. A typical ulcer is oval and about 3–4 mm in diameter, but some may be up to 2 cm in diameter. Its edge may be slightly raised and surrounded by erythematous tissue. The ulcer is shallow with a grey sloughing floor. Pain from the ulcer may make eating and even speaking difficult, often making the patient miserable. As the patient finds difficulty in cleaning his teeth there may be foetor oris.

The ulcers vary a great deal in shape, according to their site. On the cheeks and lips they tend to have a regular outline, but on the under surface of the tongue and the floor of the mouth they are far more irregular in outline, while in the vestibular sulci they tend to be serpiginous. Ulcers may occur singly or three to four at the same time. Generally there is some overlap, so that as one ulcer heals another may start. A spate of ulcers may occur associated with one of the precipitating factors, following which the patient may be free from ulcers for weeks or months. Alternatively the patient may never be free from ulcers.

Healing may start after five days, but can be delayed for up to two weeks, especially if the ulcer is persistently traumatized. Once healing starts, the ulcer usually becomes less painful. There may be some associated submandibular lymph-node tenderness, but rarely frank, palpable lymphadenopathy. The ulcer heals by epithelization from the margins and leaves a small erythematous area of new mucosa which fades in a few days. No scar remains after an aphthous ulcer has healed, provided the ulcer remains superficial and is not aggravated by trauma, medicaments or infection.

Major aphthous ulcers (often called a periadenitis-type ulcer): Ulcers are usually single and protracted in their course. In most cases there is a history of this type of ulceration, but isolated ulcers do occur in patients with a history of aphthous type ulceration. A large, deep ulcer slowly develops with raised margins which are erythematous and shiny, indicating that there is considerable oedema. The floor of the ulcer is covered with a grey slough and an indurated base may be palpated. Usually there is a definite submandibular lymphadenopathy and the patient may feel ill, with slight fever. The ulcer is extremely painful and may persist for as long as six weeks. When the ulcer eventually heals, it does so with scar formation. A cobblestone appearance may be seen in the mucosa of the lip, due to multiple ulcers healing with scar formation.

Herpetiform aphthous ulcers: A large number of small ulcers the size of a pinhead may occur in crops. As many as thirty ulcers may be seen in the mouth at the same time. At first the ulcers are discrete, surrounded by small haloes of erythema, but they may eventually coalesce into clusters. It is this similarity to herpetic lesions which has led to the use of the term 'herpetiform'.

In spite of their small size, these ulcers can be painful and can make the patient's mouth very uncomfortable, due to their large number. Healing is much quicker than with the other type of ulcer and the whole cycle may take only three to four days, but by the time this has happened there are many new ulcers. It is a very persistent condition which can be most depressing to patients in its resistance to treatment.

Differential diagnosis and investigation

Usually there is little difficulty in arriving at a diagnosis from the history, even if the ulcers have healed by the time the patient presents. Cyclical neutropenia may produce a single ulcer of the oral mucosa; this can quickly be excluded by the white cell count. Herpangina produces ulcers on the soft palate and pharynx. The Coxsackie group A viruses can often be isolated from throat washings and serological tests for the virus confirm the diagnosis. There seems little value in investigating for herpes simplex virus in the herpetiform aphthous ulcers.

Major aphthae, by their appearance, persistence and lymph-adenopathy, may mimic a squamous-cell carcinoma. A biopsy will confirm the diagnosis, but the biopsy site will be very sore for a considerable time.

Erythema multiforme and drug reactions occasionally present with recurrent ulceration which is difficult to distinguish on the basis of the history and clinical examination.

Enquiry should be made as to ocular, genital and skin lesions to exclude Behçet's and Reiter's syndromes. A blood picture should always be obtained and a serum iron estimation. Any suggestion of macrocytic anaemia should lead to full haematological investigation.

In cases where gastrointestinal symptoms are prominent or coeliac disease is suspected then, through the good offices of a gastroenterologist, investigation, including jejunal biopsy, may be arranged.

Treatment

Iron, folate or vitamin B_{12}, where indicated, are most reliably associated with a beneficial effect, but for the non-deficient patient, in the majority by 4:1, treatment is only marginally beneficial and so many different treatments have been tried in an attempt to finds a successful remedy for a common malady. Very few of the treatment regimes have been subjected to properly controlled clinical trials. Thus most of the success claimed for various treatments is purely subjective, generally based on the patient's claiming some relief from a particular preparation. There is no doubt that some patients are not happy unless they are given some form of treatment, but the majority of patients eventually learn that there is no real cure and resign themselves to living with their affliction.

Evaluation of treatment: Cooke, by the introduction of the 'ulcer-day unit', made the assessment of double-blind trials possible. Under this scheme the patient is taught to examine his own mouth once a day for ulcers. Each ulcer counts as one unit for each day it is present. A total can be made for one month and a comparison made between treatment and a placebo. This assessment does not take into consideration the severity of individual ulcers or the external environmental factors, but even so, it is the best measure available.

Current treatments: As none is totally effective, there are still a large number of current remedies with their various advocates. A summary of the main lines of treatment will be given.

1. TOPICAL ANTISEPTICS AND ANAESTHETICS: The rationale behind this line of treatment is that even if the condition cannot be cured, at least the lesions can be kept clean and the pain lessened while the condition lasts. This may well be achieved, but if too strong a preparation is used, healing will be retarded. Cases are seen in which the ulcer has become an area of chemical necrosis. Although there are a number of expensive proprietary preparations, none has any advantage over phenol and alkaline mouthwash BPC (collut. phenol alk BPC), which contains 3 per cent phenol, 3 per cent potassium hydroxide and 1 per cent amaranth. Fifteen ml are used in 100 ml (half a tumblerful or ¼ pint) of warm water. This at best gives the patient relief to start a meal, makes the mouth feel clean and is safe and cheap. Alternatively, benzalkonium lozenges BPC or benzocaine compound lozenges BPC can be used for limited periods, but even these well-tried preparations can cause a mucosal reaction if used for prolonged periods.

2. ANTIBIOTIC MOUTHWASHES: Claims have been made that a 2·5 per cent tetracycline mouth wash is effective if used qds (made by emptying the contents of one 250 mg tetracycline capsule into 100 ml of warm water, or better still, by adding the equivalent dose of tetracycline suspension to warm water). These claims have been put forward mainly for the herpetiform type of ulcer. Personal experience has in no way confirmed them and would, in fact, suggest that any success is purely due to the ulcers' healing in less than five days.

3. TOPICAL STEROIDS: Since Cooke initially showed that lozenges containing 2·5 mg of hydrocortisone hemisuccinate reduced the ulcer-day units, many topical steroids have been tried. The rationale is that they suppress the inflammatory reaction, which makes the ulcer more comfortable. It has been suggested that the steroid suppresses the local auto-immune reaction and allows healing. After the initial therapeutic euphoria which these preparations produced among eager doctors and dentists hoping for an effective treatment, clinical trials are now casting doubt on their efficacy. Hydrocortisone hemisuccinate lozenges 2·5 mg qds (Corland Pellets) gave place to 0·1 per cent triamcinolone in an emollient dental base (Adcortyl-A in Orabase) applied qds. Evaluation shows that even the stronger steroids are only marginally effective and one case of suprarenal suppression has been demonstrated. It is as well to remember that all the steroid applied topically in the mouth is absorbed, either through the oral mucosa or swallowed and absorbed through the alimentary mucosa.

Carbenoxolone sodium, which is a steroid-like substance, has been used in the treatment of peptic ulcers. Some patients claim relief when a 2 per cent solution is applied in an adherent base (Bioral Gel).

4. PROTECTING THE ULCER WHILE IT HEALS: In theory this would seem reasonable and sodium carboxymethylcellulose (Orabase) has been devised for this purpose, but clinical trials have shown that it may have little, if any, effect on the healing of aphthous ulcers.

5. OESTROGEN/PROGESTERONE PREPARATIONS: Bishop has shown that there is a group of women of childbearing age who suffer from aphthous ulcers which occur maximally premenstrually. These patients often suffer from dysmenorrhoea. When oestrogen/progesterone preparations are given as part of the treatment of their dysmenorrhoea, it is remarkable how many have a remission of their aphthous ulcers. A number of patients have been seen personally who date their remission of aphthous ulcers from commencement of oestrogen/progesterone preparations either for gynaecological reasons or as means of birth control.

6. LEVAMISOLE: A trial of azathioprine lozenges (immunosuppressant) proved ineffective and more recently levamisole which stimulates cellular immunity has been used. In a preliminary trial it produced improvement in ulcer-days in 64 per cent of patients used in a dose of 150 mg 2 days per week.

Treatments to be avoided

The old custom of cauterizing aphthous ulcers has fortunately almost died a natural death. Application of such substances as neat phenol will no doubt take the sting out of aphthous ulcers by virtue of killing the tissue, but leaves a necrotic mass which will take longer to heal. The same can be said for the use of a silver nitrate stick. Attempts to precipitate proteins to form a protective coat by the use of astringents, such as zinc chloride or sulphate and alum, are both painful and ineffective. Gentian violet does little harm, but is messy and also ineffective. In desperation, some practitioners use virtually any oral preparation in an attempt to find some suitable remedy. It is easy to condemn this in print, but when faced with a patient who has tried every known remedy and is demanding treatment, a non-scientific approach can be excused. Quite often it is remarkable what patients will claim gives them relief—antihistamines, vitamins and tranquillizers have all been tried, but with little success.

Patients should not be encouraged to subject themselves to dietary restrictions in an attempt to find initiating factors. It is true that when active ulcers are present in the mouth, citrus fruits may cause considerable pain, but they should not be excluded from the diet when the patient is symptom-free.

Behçet's Syndrome

Introduction

This was well described in ophthalmological literature before Behçet's first paper in 1937, in which he described a triple symptom complex of anterior uveitis with oral and genital ulceration. Descriptions had also appeared in the dermatological literature but concerned orogenital ulceration seen in women, without ocular involvement. Some of these cases might have been pemphigoid, however, as the 'triple symptom complex' of Behçet is rare in women.

Aetiology

This is thought to be infective (a virus is postulated) but no specific agent is known. It has also been suggested that there is an auto-immune basis for the disease and the evidence is now impressive. There are no specific features of the oral or other ulcers on histological examination.

Clinical features

Men are affected at least ten times more frequently than women, most cases occurring between the ages of 20 and 40 years. There is a chronic intermittent course with high incidence of blindness as a permanent sequela. Death is rare, but may occur in those with nervous system involvement.

In the mouth there is intermittent oral ulceration. The ulcers are non-specific and indistinguishable from aphthae (either major or minor) but tend to persist for up to one month.

Ulcers also occur on the shaft or glans of the penis and may extend on to the scrotal skin. They are shallow and oval with clearcut margins.

Severe anterior uveitis proceeding to hypopyon (pus in the anterior chamber of the eye) occurs in 80 per cent of cases. The uveitis is intermittent and blindness may supervene.

The skin may show erythema nodosum in 20 per cent of cases and erythema multiforme in half that number. The skin also shows a curious reaction to trauma: at the site of a pinprick or scratch, ulceration typical of Behçet's may follow. This susceptibility to trauma probably accounts for the high incidence of superficial purulent infections of the skin (pyoderma) noted in 30 per cent of cases.

A non-suppurative arthritis occurs in a third of cases and in a minority, perhaps 20 per cent, nervous system lesions are present. These are mainly subtentorial (the cerebellum, brain stem and spinal cord being involved) and death may occur in these, the most severe cases.

Treatment

This is symptomatic. Topical steroids are used for oral lesions. Eye involvement is best managed by an ophthalmologist with steroids, antibiotics and mydriatics.

Systemic steroids may be used in the most severe cases, but the results are disappointing.

Reiter's Syndrome

Introduction

Reiter described his syndrome in 1916 as a triad of arthritis, urethritis and conjunctivitis complicating a form of dysentery, but it had previously been noted by Benjamin Brodie in 1818.

It is now most commonly seen as a 'complication' (in about 50 per cent) of non-specific urethritis. This latter is thought to be, at least in some cases, due to *Mycoplasma hominis* infection and transmission is venereal. Abroad the disease is still seen as described by Reiter following dysentery which may be amoebic or bacillary in origin.

Aetiology

Modern evidence suggests that (as first noted by Reiter) the primary exciting factor in the disease is a shigella infection. The *urethritis* is probably part of the altered immunological response like the mucosal lesions, uveitis and arthritis. The role of *Mycoplasma hominis* as the aetiological agent in the urethritis is less than certain. The response pattern which 'is' the syndrome is strongly conditioned by genetic factors—HLA B27 being identifiable in 65 per cent of these patients but only 10 per cent of controls.

Clinical features

This disease occurs much more commonly in men in the 20–40 age group. There is an acute onset and arthritis and urethritis are the most striking features. The large weight-bearing joints are principally involved; suppuration does not occur.

Conjunctivitis occurs in 50 per cent of cases, but rarely a relapsing uveitis develops which may lead to blindness. In 10 per cent of cases small non-specific ulcers, identical to aphthae, occur in the mouth.

Ulcers on the penis, rather like those of Behçet's syndrome, occur in 25 per cent of cases. A 'sterile' mucopurulent urethral discharge is present in all cases and usually antedates other symptoms. The urethritis is characterized by frequency of micturition and dysuria.

In a few cases an unusual skin eruption occurs which is characterized by hyperkeratosis of the palms and soles; it is called keratodermia blennorrhagica.

Rare complications include a peripheral neuropathy and myocarditis. The disease usually burns out over a month or two, but several relapses may occur.

Chronic sacro-iliitis and spondylitis may persist and be associated with relapsing uveitis, but with that exception, complete recovery is the rule.

Investigations

The ESR is greatly elevated at the onset. Concurrent gonococcal infection is not unusual and must be excluded by examination of the urethral discharge.

Treatment

Tetracycline is usually administered for a two-week course. Aspirin is necessary to control the pain (arthralgia) and later physiotherapy is instituted to rehabilitate the limbs. Uveitis should be treated by an ophthalmologist.

Human Lymphatic Antigen (HLA) and Oral Disease

In man the major 'transplantation' antigen system is named human lymphatic antigen (HLA) and there is some link between the presence of particular genes of this system and susceptibility to some diseases. There is a link between this gene group, Behçet's and Reiter's syndromes.

In this system there are 4 loci with 20 antigens at the A and B loci, 5 at the C and 8 at the D loci.

The strongest association is between ankylosing spondylitis and HLA B27 but this antigen is also associated with Reiter's syndrome, acute uveitis and Still's disease, i.e.

	HLA B27
Controls	5–10%
Ankylosing spondylitis	95%
Reiter's syndrome	65%
Uveitis	27%
Still's disease	25%

The risk of any individual with HLA B27 developing spondylitis is small but it is clear that the presence of this particular gene renders its possessor uniquely responsive to an unidentified environmental agent. Whether it is other genetic variability or 'trigger' differences that produce the variable response (arthritis, uveitis, spondylitis) is not clear. Further there is an almost equally strong relationship between HLA B5 and Behçet's syndrome in Japan, but not in Europe.

Here again the likelihood is that an extrinsic agent acts to elicit a particular disease response in some way conditioned by the genetic factor.

A more complex relationship exists between the HLA system and reactivity to gluten (gluten-sensitive enteropathy, coeliac disease) and dermatitis herpetiformis. Here the relationship is with A1/B8/DW3, and again the genetic endowment appears to predispose to the special reactivity to gluten. A1/B8 is the commonest haplotype in caucasians.

The HLA system thus has a relationship with some of the types of oral ulceration outlined in this chapter. The apparent non-relationship with aphthous ulceration indicates the probable multiple aetiology of that disorder.

Necrotizing Sialometaplasia

A clinicopathological entity of mysterious aetiology which is often a cause of diagnostic confusion.

Pathogenesis

The primary abnormality seems to develop in the minor salivary glands which necrose while ductal epithelium undergoes squamous metaplasia.

The onset of the disorder is quite abrupt and eventual healing takes several weeks which suggests some infective agent *or* primary antigenic variation (chimaerism) in the damaged epithelium.

Clinical features

The patient may first note a painful swelling but generally presents when ulceration supervenes at about 1 week. The lesion always occurs in the pad of mucous glands lateral to the midline at the posterior end of the hard palate, generally closer to the gingival margin than the midline.

The ulcer is deep with clear-cut edges and a coagulum in the base, while the surrounding tissue is inflamed and somewhat oedematous. It is generally round or oval in shape.

Eventually, after several weeks (up to 6), the ulcer heals by secondary intention.

Diagnosis

The condition must be distinguished from salivary neoplasms which is generally not difficult as the latter cause more swelling and less ulceration. On the basis of the history alone squamous-cell carcinoma may be suspected but the clinical appearances rule this out, and this is a very unusual site for such a carcinoma. Biopsy is mandatory if any doubt as to diagnosis remains in the clinician's mind, otherwise nothing need be done but observe till healing is complete.

Agranulocytosis and Neutropenia

Similar oral lesions may occur when normal mature white cells are lacking for any reason. Leukaemia (*see* Chapter 8) is one of a number of causes of such problems and in many cases bacterial invasion appears to be the proximate cause of ulceration (*see* Chapter 4).

Agranulocytosis means literally absence of granulocytes while leucopenia implies pathological reduction in the numbers of white cells. The terms are often used loosely, interchangeably.

Many cases are due to drugs—either by a direct toxic action on the marrow or by immunological mechanisms affecting circulating cells. Other cases are due to marrow diseases. Such patients may present with oral ulceration which *initially* is associated with irregular inflammatory patches of mucosa. The ulceration, initially shallow, may progress to extensive necrotic lesions but some healing and recurrence may occur.

Diagnosis

This can only be effected by examination of the blood and thence detailed history and further investigation as indicated.

Treatment

Scrupulous oral hygiene is important and either bactericidal antibiotics or metronidazole may be helpful. If these are used it may be helpful to maintain an oral flora of lactobacilli by use of yoghourt. Ultimately the prognosis depends upon that for the underlying disease and obviously treatment must be directed to the cause.

Bibliography

Barile M. F. et al. (1963) L-form of bacteria isolated from recurrent aphthous stomatitis lesions. *Oral Surg.* 16, 1395.

Bishop P. M. F. et al. (1967) Oestrogen treatment of recurrent aphthous mouth ulcers. *Lancet* 1, 1345.

Browne R. M. et al. (1968) Topical triamcinolone acetonide in recurrent aphthous stomatitis. *Lancet* 1, 565.

Challacombe S. J. et al. (1977) Haematological features and differentiation of recurrent oral ulceration. *Br. J. Oral Surg.* 15, 37.

Cooke B. E. D. and Armitage P. (1960) Recurrent Mikulicz's aphthae treated with topical hydrocortisone hemisuccinate sodium. *Br. Med. J.* 1, 764

Dolby A. E. (1969) Recurrent aphthous ulceration, effect of sera and peripheral blood lymphocytes upon oral epithelial tissue culture cells. *Immunology* 17, 709.

Dolby A. E. (1970) Mikulicz recurrent oral aphthae: the effect of anti-lymphocytic serum upon the in vitro cytotoxicity of lymphocytes from patients for oral epithelial cells. *Clin. Exp. Immunol.* 7, 681.

Ferguson R. et al. (1976) Jejunal mucosal abnormalities in patients with recurrent aphthous ulceration. *Br. Med. J.* 1, 11.

Graykowski E. A. et al. (1966) Recurrent aphthous stomatitis. *JAMA* 196, 637.

Lehner T. (1964) Recurrent aphthous stomatitis and autoimmunity. *Lancet* 2, 1154.

Lehner T. (1968) Auto-immunity in oral disease with specific reference to recurrent oral ulceration. *Proc. R. Soc. Med.* 61, 515.

Lehner T. (1977) Oral ulceration and Behçet's syndrome. *Gut* 18, 491.

Luzard-Baptista M. J. (1975) Aspects of the fine anatomy of aphthous stomatitis. *Oral Surg.* 39, 239.

MacPhee I. T. et al. (1968) Use of steroids in treatment of aphthous ulceration. *Br. Med. J.* 1, 147.

Medical Annual (1975) Tropical sprue. 339.

Oliver R. T. D. (1977) Histocompatability antigens and human disease. *Br. J. Hosp. Med.* 17, 449.

Ship I. I. et al. (1960) Recurrent aphthous ulcerations and recurrent herpes labialis in a professional school student population. *Oral Surg.* 13, 1191, 1317, 1438; 14, 30.

Sircus W. et al. (1957) Recurrent aphthous ulceration of the mouth. *Q. J. Med.* **26,** 235.

Williams B. D. and Lehner T. (1977) Immune complexes in Behçet's syndrome and recurrent oral ulceration. *Br. Med. J.* **1,** 1387.

Wray D. et al. (1975) Recurrent aphthae: treatment with vitamin B_{12}, folic acid and iron. *Br. Med. J.* **1,** 490.

Chapter 2

Vesiculobullous Lesions

In this chapter are described the diseases which have in common the presence of oral ulceration which follows the breakdown of vesicles or bullae.

Vesicles and bullae are due to the accumulation of fluid either within the epithelium or between the epithelium and the lamina propria (or dermis of the skin). Bullae are large and vesicles small.

In the mouth both bullae and vesicles very quickly burst to leave ulcers which usually have peripheral tags of epithelium which are the remnants of the roof of the blister.

Herpes simplex infection is by far the *commonest* cause of vesiculobullous lesions in the mouth whilst zoster and Coxsackie infections—hand, foot and mouth disease and herpangina, are also recognized aetiological agents. Apart from these, which will be considered in Chapter 3, the following will be described here:

1. Epidermolysis bullosae.
2. Pemphigus
3. Pemphigoid.
4. Erythema multiforme.
5. Amyloidosis.
6. Dermatitis herpetiformis.

Epidermolysis Bullosae

This is an inherited disorder of which there are two subgroups: a simple form inherited as a Mendelian dominant in which intra-epithelial bullae occur and a more severe dystrophic form, inherited as a recessive and associated with subepithelial bullae. Both are rare. The bullae in each case are an abnormal response to trauma, which may be minimal in the case of the simple variety.

Pathogenesis

In addition to the bullae described above, a degeneration of the elastic tissue of the dermis has also been noted in the dystrophic variety. The underlying biochemical abnormality which is due to the abnormal gene and is the proximate cause of the observed lesions is, however, unknown.

Clinical features

In the dystrophic type, bullae appear soon after birth both on the skin and in the mouth due to suckling. Rarely the features appear in an older patient.

The bullae heal slowly and with scarring. The scars on the skin are paper-thin and pale. If the patient survives, hypoplasia of the teeth may be noted. An exceptional case with extra-articular ankylosis of the temporomandibular joint due to scarring in the mouth has been reported.

Severe disability is usual and early death follows, but in patients who survive a progressive reduction in liability to bulla formation occurs.

In the simple form, bullae follow obvious trauma but are not followed by scarring. Lesions of the mouth are *exceptional*. In such cases, however, the careful avoidance of trauma in the mouth is essential.

Diagnosis is based on the family history and the association of the bullae with trauma. There is no effective treatment.

Pemphigus

This is a disease characterized by a lack of cohesion of the prickle cell layer, with the presence of degenerate acantholytic cells of stratified squamous epithelium. Recurrent intra-epithelial bullae occur and the disease is progressive; prior to the introduction of steroids it was almost always fatal.

Previous to the work of Civatte (1943) and Lever (1953), all bullous lesions were designated as pemphigus of one form or another, i.e. pemphigus neonatorum or 'benign' pemphigus. It is now appreciated that true pemphigus as defined above is a specific disease and must be distinguished from a group of bullous lesions which may imitate it. Principal among these is *pemphigoid*, which is characterized by the presence of *subepithelial bullae*, without acantholysis, in the elderly patient.

There are four clinical varieties of pemphigus—pemphigus vulgaris, the common form which is described, pemphigus vegetans, pemphigus foliaceus and pemphigus erythematosus (Senear–Usher syndrome).

Pathology

The typical lesion of pemphigus is a bulla. This results from the lack of cohesion of the prickle cells. Typically the weakest line in the epithelium is at the junction of the basal cell and prickle cell layers and here splits occur. These splits may extend over a very wide area and an exudate of plasma enters to produce a flaccid bulla.

The abnormal epithelial cells lining the bullae may be demonstrated in histological section or by smears and are termed acantholytic or Tzanck cells. These are small rounded cells with a rim of condensed eosinophilic cytoplasm and pyknotic (degenerating) nuclei.

Aetiology and pathogenesis

The disease is acquired but the aetiology is unknown; it appears to be common in Jews. It has been thought to be infective and lately, auto-immune. It is possible in all cases to demonstrate an antibody which is directed toward some component of the structures uniting the epithelial cells. In association with lesions the antibody is found coating the cells and complement is fixed thereto.

The explicit reason for the development of the antibody is not clear but the pathogenesis of the lesions is clearly immunological.

Clinical features

The onset is usually between the ages of 30 and 50 years and the sex incidence is equal. The patient may present with oral ulceration; if not the initial symptom, this commonly develops soon after the onset. The oral ulceration follows the rupture of bullae and an intelligent patient may note the transient bullous stage. These erosions are painful and tend to extend progressively after their initial appearance. Examination reveals large irregular erosions with tags of epithelium at the edges. Rarely a collapsed bulla may be seen. This looks like a piece of wrinkled tissue-paper applied to the mucosa, which on being lifted up reveals the erosion (the floor of the bulla) beneath. Very rarely a bulla may be seen and a careful search should be made for one.

In cases with these features, the mucosa should be gently pressed and a lateral force applied. If the epithelium splits and the superficial layers slide under the finger, Nikolsky's sign is said to be present (Pyotr Vasilyevich Nikolsky, Russian dermatologist, born 1855). It is diagnostic of pemphigus in the absence of epidermolysis bullosae.

The skin manifestations of pemphigus are the appearance of bullae (usually described by the patient as blisters). These appear spontaneously and are relatively fragile; thus they burst. They also extend progressively until large areas of skin may be denuded and weeping.

It is most important to establish the diagnosis at the earliest possible time and oral manifestations may be the only features for up to a year in over half the patients. Thus in any case suspected of being pemphigus the following investigations should be performed.

1. The base of the bulla should be scraped and the cells placed on a slide for cytological examination for acantholytic cells.

2. A lesion, preferably a fresh bulla, should be excised or biopsied.

3. The skin should be examined completely.

4. The ESR should be estimated.

The progress of the disease is inexorable in the absence of treatment. Oral lesions make eating difficult and large areas of the skin may be covered with bullae from which fluid weeps. Hypoalbuminaemia develops with a reactive rise in the globulins. Death occurs in 100 per cent of cases in the absence of treatment.

Treatment

As soon as the diagnosis is established, the patient should be admitted to hospital for treatment which consists of prednisone in doses large enough to control symptoms and signs. Initially this may be 60–80 mg per day (or more) but later is reduced to a maintenance dose which is varied according to control. Dosage is such that features of iatrogenic Cushing's syndrome are frequently produced.

An easily assimilated high protein diet is indicated if the serum albumin is low. With widespread skin lesions nursing may prove an intractable problem.

On such a regime recovery may occur in 2–3 years and it may be possible to withdraw steroids, but some patients have to be kept on small maintenance doses. The overall mortality is approximately halved by steroid therapy.

The other rare variants of pemphigus described above are relatively benign and in only a few cases are oral lesions a feature.

Pemphigoid

(*Synonyms:* Benign mucous membrane pemphigoid, Benign mucous membrane pemphigus, Ocular pemphigus.)

This disorder of the aged is characterized by the appearance of sub-epithelial bullae on mucosae (mouth and genitalia) and especially the conjunctiva, less commonly on the skin. It runs a relapsing course, but is invariably benign in the sense that it does not lead to death. The unusual occurrence of blindness is the most severe complication.

Aetiology

Unknown, but it is possible to demonstrate fixation of immunoglobulin to the basement membrane in relationship to lesions. There appear, however, to be no circulating antibodies.

Pathology

Subepithelial bullae are present. Fluid accumulates between the epidermis and dermis (or lamina propria). There is adjacent chronic cell infiltration. There are no degenerative epithelial changes, such as acantholysis, as found in pemphigus. The roof of the bulla is the whole epidermis and so the bullae tend not to rupture as they do in pemphigus, neither do they enlarge after formation.

Clinical features

The disease is found in the elderly, hence being rare before the age of 50 and most common after 70 years. It is more common in females.

The eyes are usually prominently involved and typically are affected first. There are shallow conjunctival erosions which heal with scarring. Considerable contraction of the conjunctival fornices follows and adhesions may develop (symblepharon). Vascularization of the conjunctival cornea and later keratinization may lead to visual disturbances. Scarring of the lacrimal ducts may lead to xerophthalmia.

Bullous lesions are almost invariable in the mouth; although stronger than in pemphigus, they usually burst here to leave large irregular ulcers which are relatively painless. These heal very slowly and the site of old lesions may be revealed by lacy fibrosis. Similar anogenital lesions occur.

The skin is minimally involved, usually on the perineum and around the mouth. Bullae and collapsed crusted lesions are seen. The scalp may be similarly affected.

The disease is not serious, but has considerable nuisance value. On rare occasions there may be an underlying visceral carcinoma.

Treatment

Topical steroids are the treatment of choice in the mouth and eye. Systemic steroids give disappointing results. The ocular lesions should be managed by an ophthalmologist.

Erythema Multiforme

(*Synonyms:* Erythema multiforme exudativum, Ectodermosis erosiva pluriorificialis, Stevens–Johnson syndrome.)

This is a syndrome of multiple aetiology and with a wide spectrum of clinical features. The most severe form with acute onset is termed erythema multiforme exudativum. The more common minor form is usually manifested by a cutaneous eruption but may occur as an enanthem in the mouth. Oral and cutaneous lesions may occur together in the minor form.

In about a third of all cases there are recurrences, usually two or three.

The disease was described by Von Hebra in 1866, the severe form as erythema multiforme exudativum, the minor form as erythema multiforme. The severe form was redescribed by Stevens and Johnson in 1922.

Aetiology

The origin of the syndrome is probably in several underlying mechanisms. Drug allergy is known to produce it, especially long-acting sulphonamides, penicillin and barbiturates. Several cases have been associated with infection with *Mycoplasma pneumoniae* (Eaton agent), the cause of the condition often termed 'primary atypical pneumonia'. In many cases no cause can be discovered.

Major Form

Clinical features

The patient is usually a child or a young adult. There is a skin eruption with conjunctivitis and lesions of the mouth and upper respiratory tract. There is a fairly acute onset; initially the patient is not very ill, but may become quite prostrated by the end of a week or two.

Mouth

There is a diffuse inflammation of the mouth, little vesicles occur but usually widespread erosions are seen which have a red, velvety base and bleed freely. The lips are most severely involved and extensive crusting occurs; the mucocutaneous junction is obscured. The lips and other opposed epithelial surfaces may be crusted together at night. Eating and examination of the mouth prove painful, such lesions also occur through the upper respiratory tract. Epistaxis is common. Dysphagia is severe and tracheitis may occur. Extension of the disease into the lungs with pneumonia may occur and naturally contributes to the mortality.

On the skin, erythema multiforme means what it says and an extensive erythematous or macular rash is present. 'Iris' target lesions with a central bulla which breaks down to crust are typical. The hands and feet and flexural surfaces are usually most involved.

In the eyes there is first a diffuse conjunctivitis which is commonly secondarily infected to produce corneal ulceration and possible panophthalmitis.

Urogenital inflammation and ulceration is common. An exudative arthritis may occur. Pneumonia, nephritis and myocarditis may occur in severe cases and may cause death, or the patient may die of toxaemia without apparent visceral involvement.

Investigations

The ESR is raised and leucocytosis is usual. Nasopharyngeal or cough swabs should be taken in an attempt to isolate *Mycoplasma pneumoniae*. Serum should also be taken and compared with serum taken three weeks later for titre of complement-fixing antibodies to *Mycoplasma pneumoniae*.

Minor Form: The features described above may occur without any systemic involvement, either with skin involvement or skin and oral involvement or in the mouth only.

There is no fever, no prostration and the local manifestations are similar but not as marked as in the major forms.

Treatment

In the mouth topical steroids may be employed. In the most severe cases systemic steroids and supportive treatment are necessary. If there is evidence of infection with *Mycoplasma*, either tetracycline 250 mg qds or dimethylchlortetracycline 300 mg bd should be given.

Amyloidosis

Cutaneous and oral bullae may be the presenting clinical feature of primary amyloidosis.

Aetiology and pathogenesis

The aetiology of primary amyloidosis is unknown but the deposits of amyloid are thought to be due to abnormal function of the immunoglobulin forming cells. Amyloid is an insoluble protein which in primary amyloidosis is deposited in the heart, kidneys, liver, gut, nerves and skin. The bullae result from shearing of intradermal amyloid deposits which apparently induce weaknesses in the dermis and associated vasculature.

Clinical features

Skin involvement is usually manifested by papular infiltration in the head and neck accompanied by petechial haemorrhage. Oral features include macroglossia which however only occurs in 25–50 per cent of cases, submucosal plaques and petechial haemorrhage.

Oral bullae, when they occur, appear to result from minor trauma and in this condition are filled with bloodstained fluid (or apparently blood only). These 'bloodblisters' are persistently recurrent and each heals in a few days. Cutaneous bullae are by comparison rare.

Primary amyloidosis is notoriously difficult to diagnose. As far as the oral features are concerned bloodblisters of the oral mucosa are not uncommon especially in the elderly so further investigation is only indicated if the patient has other suggestive features such as unexplained skin lesions, heart, gut, liver or renal failure or peripheral neuropathy.

The mucosal lesions at least provide a target for biopsy. In trying to confirm a diagnosis of amyloid in the absence of mucosal lesions, biopsy of the tongue and lower labial vestibular mucosa may provide the answer but less certainly than rectal biopsy. The biopsy material must be stained with Congo red and examined under polarized light, or with Thioflavine-T and examined under ultraviolet light.

Dermatitis Herpetiformis

This is a cutaneous eruption due to gluten sensitivity and associated with jejunal mucosal abnormalities. There is rarely any clinical evidence of malabsorption and oral lesions are very rare.

Clinical features

The skin, especially of the lower limbs, develops recurrent subepidermal tense bullae of which the main characteristic is extreme itchiness. The eruption is long standing and progressive changes in local skin pigmentation (excessive or reduced) follow.

In the mouth, bullae (which, as always, rupture readily) have been reported. They do not occur, apparently, unless skin lesions are extremely well marked.

Bibliography

Brandtzaeg P. (1964) Erythema multiforme exudativum. *Odontol. Tidsk.* **12**, 363.

Cooke B. E. D. (1960) The diagnosis of bullous lesions affecting the oral mucosa. *Br. Dent. J.* **109**, 83, 131.

Harris M. (1967) Pemphigoid (Benign mucous membrane pemphigus). *Br. J. Oral Surg.* **5**, 42.

Keith D. A. (1972) Oral features of primary amyloidosis. *Br. J. Oral Surg.* **10**, 107.

Lubarsch O. (1929) Zur Kenntnis ungewöhnlicher Amyloidablagerungen. *Virchow's Arch.* (*Pathol. Anat.*) **271**, 867.

Northover J. M. A. et al. (1972) Bullous lesions of the skin and mucous membranes in primary amyloidosis. *Postgrad. Med. J.* **48**, 351.

Russotto S. B. and Ship I. I. (1971) Oral manifestations of dermatitis herpetiformis. *Oral Surg.* **31**, 42.

Shklar G. (1968) Erosive and bullous lesions of lichen planus. *Arch. Dermatol.* **97**, 411.

Shklar G., Meyer I. and Zacarian S. A. (1969) Oral lesions in bullous pemphigoid. *Arch. Dermatol.* **99**, 663.

Sneddon I. B. (1968) Immunological aspects of pemphigus and pemphigoid. *Br. J. Dermatol.* **80**, 410.

Chapter 3

Oral Infections (Viral)

Viral infections attacking the oral mucosa and producing vesiculobullous lesions and ulcers, apart from the enanthem of measles and smallpox, are due to two groups of agents, namely, herpes viruses and the Coxsackie group. In addition, virally-induced hypoplasias will be considered here.
1. Herpes simplex infections.
2. Herpes varicella–zoster infections.
3. Epstein–Barr virus (Infectious mononucleosis).
4. Coxsackie infections.
5. Measles.
6. Virally-induced epithelial hyperplasias.

Herpes Simplex Infections

Infections are characterized by a severe systemic upset during primary infection and subsequently a susceptibility to recurrent lesions, probably due to activation of latent virus in an immune host.

Aetiology and pathology

Herpes simplex virus is a cylindrical DNA-based organism about 100 μm in size but may acquire a soluble envelope which doubles the overall size. Like many viruses it is resistant to cold and may be cultured on the allantoic membrane of fertile hens eggs, tissue cultures or in experimental animals. The virus has a marked predilection to invade epithelial cells and these show characteristic cytological changes which include the development of nuclear inclusion bodies and multinucleated giant cells and cell destruction. The nuclear inclusions apparently evolve from small to large basophilic bodies which displace the chromatin peripherally. The inclusions become eosinophilic presumably after release of the infective viral particles and these eosinophilic inclusions have been termed the Lipschultz bodies. The cytological changes include the fusion

27

of infected with normal cells to produce a small syncytial mass (giant cell) with multiple nuclei. In some cases (apparently a different viral strain) multiple nuclear divisions occur without cytoplasmic division and so another form of multinucleated giant cell is produced. These cells are highly characteristic in smears of cells from herpetic lesions and have been aptly described as mulberry cells. Among the histological features of herpetic lesions cytolysis is prominent with the production of intra-epithelial vesicles. The epithelium at the base of the vesicle may be destroyed so that the vesicle is subepithelial. The cells at the periphery of the vesicle may show the features noted above but they are not prominent in histological preparations. *Herpes simplex* infection is associated with a brisk antibody response.

Clinical features

The many and varied clinical features of *Herpes simplex* infections may be grouped as follows:

- *a.* Primary infection
  - i. *Gingivostomatitis.*
  - ii. Dermal, ocular and genital.
  - iii. Encephalomyelitis.
- *b.* Recurrent infection (or activation)
  - i. Herpes labialis.
  - ii. Recurrent oral herpes.
  - iii. Dendritic corneal ulcer.

i. *Acute herpetic gingivostomatitis:* Although in the majority of cases the primary infection is subclinical or asymptomatic, its most frequent clinical expression is a severe gingivostomatitis. The disease is more common in children between the ages of 1 and 10 years but is not infrequent in adults. There is an acute onset with high fever and malaise, the patient is fractious and off his food. Marked submandibular and upper deep cervical lymphadenopathy is present. The oral mucosa is diffusely inflamed and the gingivae acutely inflamed, swollen and bleed readily. The characteristic lesions are vesicles which occur all over the oral mucosa but particularly on the palate adjacent to the deciduous molars (or in adults the premolars) and on the gingival margin. The vesicles are very thin walled, appearing as little drops of dew on the mucosa which rapidly break down to form shallow painful concave ulcers of 1–2 mm in diameter on top of small conical elevations rather like moon craters. It is most unusual to see a case without an unbroken vesicle which points to the diagnosis, but in adults the ulcerated lesions may be few and larger than in children and indistinguishable from aphthae although the history is usually sufficient to distinguish the two. The diagnosis is established by scraping the floor of an unbroken vesicle (after removal of the roof) and examination of the cells microscopically. It is most unusual not to see the typical cells described above and their presence establishes the diagnosis (identical cells are seen in chickenpox and zoster, but these two are quite obvious clinically). Further proof of the diagnosis may be obtained (although retrospectively) by virus isolation or estimation of antibody titres. For the latter, blood is required initially and 21 days later, when a substantial rise in titre is demonstrated.

TREATMENT: Although the disease is self-limited and remits spontaneously in about 14 days, considerable symptomatic relief may be obtained by giving elixir tetracycline 250 mg qds (for adults) rinsed around the mouth after meals. For children elixir of erythromycin is used.

ii. *Herpetic dermal, ocular and genital lesions:* Although rare as primary manifestations, extensive skin lesions may occur in infants with eczema (Kaposi's varicelliform eruption) in which an extensive vesicular rash develops and may prove fatal. Among adults a primary infection may lead to a crop of vesicles on the face around the mouth or nose or genitalia which resemble those of recurrent lesions. The ocular lesions appear as a vesicular conjunctivitis.

iii. *Encephalomyelitis:* Exceptionally virus may be implicated in aetiology of aseptic meningitis (which is benign) or encephalitis (which is frequently fatal).

Recurrent infections: Up to 90 per cent of adults have circulating neutralizing antibody in spite of which about one-third of the population are subject to recurrent herpetic lesions. These are thought to be due to latent virus which is activated by a local or systemic disturbance upsetting the delicate balance between virus and epithelial cells. They may, however, be due to re-infection. In either event the lesions are localized, contained apparently, by the immunity of the host.

i. *Herpes labialis* (herpes febrilis, fever blisters): These lesions occur as a result of local trauma, exposure to sunlight or a severe systemic disturbance, particularly a fever. The first sign is swelling of the lip with soreness and then a localized crop of vesicles form on the lip adjacent to the mucocutaneous junction. These soon break down to weep serum and crust, finally healing in 10–14 days. Unless there is secondary infection the regional lymph nodes are not enlarged. Forman has noted the frequency with which herpes labialis precedes erythema multiforme.

Recurrent herpes may occur in sites other than the lips.

ii. *Recurrent oral herpes:* On rare occasions recurrent intra-oral lesions, which may be clinically indistinguishable from aphthae, are due to herpetic infection. At each recurrence typical giant cells may be recovered from the lesions.

iii. *Recurrent ocular herpetic infection:* In the cornea leads to the 'dendritic ulcer' which is painful and dangerous. Treatment with steroids is liable to lead to perforation of the globe.

Recurrent *Herpes labialis* may be treated with topical iodoxuridine but its real value lies in the treatment of the dendritic ulcer.

Herpes Varicella–Zoster Infections

This agent causes both chickenpox and shingles and is similar in structure to the *Herpes simplex* virus. The similarity extends to the pattern of infection, there being on primary contact an acute systemic infection (chickenpox) with establishment of immunity and a localized activation of latent virus (or re-infection) in immune adults producing zoster or shingles. The pathology of epithelial lesions in chickenpox and zoster is identical to those in *Herpes simplex* infections.

Chickenpox is so infectious that 90 per cent of children suffer from it. The incubation period of 14 days is succeeded by the exanthem which evolves through 4–5 days, followed by crops of fresh lesions. Each lesion evolves from macule to papule to vesicle, which crusts and may be secondarily infected. The whole illness lasts about 14 days. The enanthem is relatively insignificant. The dangerous complications, apart from pneumonia and encephalitis, are due to secondary bacterial infections.

Herpes Zoster (shingles): This disorder principally affects the elderly and represents activation of latent virus in a sensory posterior root ganglion. The affected ganglion is inflamed and the ganglion cells show degeneration with subsequent Wallerian degeneration of their axons and dendrites. The ganglion invotved is spinal in 70 per cent of cases and cephalic in 30 per cent. Skin lesions are clinically and pathologically identical to those of chickenpox.

Clinical features

Zoster is a disease of the elderly characterized by the development of neuralgic pains which are burning or stabbing, either constant or intermittent, radiating along the course of the affected nerve. In 4–5 days they are succeeded by skin lesions over the cutaneous distribution of the sensory fibres derived from the infected ganglion. From a spinal ganglion the lesions, therefore, extend round in a narrow band from the spinal column to the midline anteriorly, which accounts for the name shingles (a girdle). Involvement of the trigeminal ganglion (the sensory ganglion of the face) leads to involvement of one or two divisions, rarely all three. The lesions may be few or extensive and accurately map out the cutaneous and mucosal distribution of the division involved. Involvement of the ophthalmic division may lead to the most-feared complication of corneal ulceration and immediate ophthalmological help is required. Nasal lesions may be extensive with weeping, crusting and perhaps epistaxis. Involvement of the maxillary division leads to lesions of the hard and soft palate and the vestibule of the upper jaw. Involvement of the mandibular division leads to the most extensive cutaneous lesions from chin to vertex. In the mouth they involve the cheek, the vestibule of the lower jaw and the tongue. In the mouth the vesicles rapidly break down to form ulcers. Cytological changes in the vesicles or ulcers are as described under herpes simplex. Secondary infection of skin lesions is quite common and healing is then followed by scarring which may be recognized and is diagnostic in cases of post-herpetic neuralgia.

Treatment

A topical antibiotic cream is useful to prevent secondary infection of skin lesions and considerable relief from oral lesions may be obtained by the use of elixir of tetracycline. Analgesics may be required. Post-herpetic neuralgia is not common but tends to occur in the very aged and remits in six months to one year being resistant even to neurosurgical attack. Zoster of the geniculate ganglion (the Ramsay–Hunt syndrome) will be considered in Chapter 19.

Epstein–Barr Virus (infectious mononucleosis)

The Epstein–Barr virus which was first isolated from cases of Burkitt's lymphoma is apparently the aetiological agent of infectious mononucleosis (glandular fever). It is a *Herpes* virus. With the recognition of the cause it is to be hoped that there will be clarification of the group of illnesses which are clinically indistinguishable from glandular fever but are not associated with a positive Paul–Bunnell test. Some of such illnesses are certainly due to toxoplasmosis, but many are of unknown aetiology.

Aetiology

There is circumstantial evidence that infectious mononucleosis is due to the EB virus. At Yale University immunofluorescent techniques and complement-fixation tests have demonstrated that patients who develop Paul–Bunnell positive glandular fever also have antibodies to the EB virus. The EB virus is a *herpes*-like virus which was cultured from lymphoblasts derived from the Burkitt's lymphoma tumours, by Epstein and Barr in 1964. Although these antibodies have been demonstrated after the clinical appearance of glandular fever in patients who did not have antibodies at previous testing, no organism has been isolated and Koch's postulates are far from complete. Patients who have antibodies demonstrate immunity to glandular fever.

Cytomegalic virus has been shown to produce Paul–Bunnell negative 'glandular fever'. Toxoplasmosis will also produce a similar syndrome. A number of other organisms have been claimed to give a similar picture by other workers. It may be that glandular fever is a syndrome that can be produced by a number of different agents.

Many interesting theories have been put forward as to how the disease is transmitted. It certainly occurs commonly in young communities of people, and the 'kissing' theory is currently most popular.

Pathology

Typical mononuclear cells are seen in the blood and may originate from the enlarged glands. The total monocyte count is increased to as much as 50 per cent of the total white cell count. There may be some increase in lymphocytes with mild depression of the granulocytes and platelets. Of the many antibodies that have been demonstrated, the most famous, and best, is the Paul–Bunnell reaction for heterophil antibodies. Claims have been made that the specific antigen is neuraminic acid. The appearance of antibodies has been shown to give a 100 per cent rise in IgM and a 50 per cent rise in IgG.

Clinical features

Infectious mononucleosis is most common in the age group 15–25 and occurs more frequently in young people living in a close community.

There can be a type of 'smouldering epidemic' where, as one patient recovers, another case occurs. Figures given for the incubation period are more traditional than factual. Subclinical attacks must be quite common if the detection of EB virus antibodies can be relied upon, as many older people have antibodies but no clinical history.

Since Sir Henry Tidy (1952) described six different clinical forms of glandular fever, it has become almost obligatory to follow suit, but it must be remembered that this is useful for ease of description, but that clinical cases will not always be so easily divided.

Juvenile Glandular Type: There is a short period of malaise followed by a glandular enlargement, which may be the first sign. Cervical nodes are most commonly involved and the enlargement may be visible as a swelling which arises in as short a time as 24 hours. The mediastinal glands may also be enlarged, but it is rare for them to cause respiratory obstruction. A sore throat is common but rarely is there any exudative tonsillitis.

Splenic enlargement is common in this group. Although the patient may have a fever, the constitutional features of the disease are usually mild and will settle in two to three weeks. Relapses are occasionally seen. This type of glandular fever is called the juvenile form because it occurs most frequently in children, but from time to time adults are subjected to attacks of glandular fever which take this form.

Adolescent Type: This is more an insidious form of the disease, with a low grade fever and mild lymphadenopathy. Often the only feature noted by the patient is a general malaise. Claims have been made that this type of the disease is more common among nurses and medical students. In these cases the diagnosis is made by the patients themselves, or it is observed at a routine medical examination.

Prolonged Febrile Type: The febrile period is variable and may be prolonged. It may even subside before glandular enlargement is noted. During the febrile phase there are no diagnostic features and investigations do not help. Serology for syphilis may be found to be temporarily positive which can cause unnecessary embarrassment. The confusion can be increased by a commonly palpable spleen and a rubelliform rash.

Anginose Type: This often presents as a membranous tonsillitis in young men. There may even be ulcers in the mouth and spongy gums which bleed easily. Accompanying these features may be a pyrexia of up to 104°F. At the junction of the hard and soft palate there may be petechial haemorrhages. In this form involvement of liver, spleen, heart, lungs and kidneys have been demonstrated. Cervical lymphadenopathy is usually a prominent feature and there may be some oedema of the face and eyelids.

Neurological manifestations

These are rare, occurring in only about 1 per cent of cases. The commonest form is an aseptic meningitis, but there may also be a polyneuritis of the Guillain–Barré type. Many other neurological features have been reported, often making the clinical picture very confusing; not even glandular enlargement can be relied upon to give a clinical lead. Recovery is usually complete from the neurological point of view, but can often be delayed.

Onset with jaundice

In these cases the clinical picture is indistinguishable from infective hepatitis. Even after liver function tests have been reported there is little to distinguish the two diseases. In cases of infective hepatitis which subsequently develop lymphadenopathy, glandular fever should be suspected.

Diagnosis

For practical purposes a positive Paul–Bunnell test is diagnostic of glandular fever, but a positive reaction may be delayed in the febrile phase, appearing when glandular enlargement is manifest.

False positives are rare but have been reported in rheumatoid arthritis and Hodgkin's disease. It is impossible to estimate the incidence of false negatives.

As glandular fever concerns a wide range of signs and symptoms the differential diagnosis is equally wide, ranging from any cause of glandular enlargement, febrile conditions with enlarged liver and spleen, jaundice, tonsillitis and aseptic meningitis. In a series reported by Fraser–Moodie oral lesions occurred in 30 per cent of cases and included a gingivostomatitis, palatal petechiae and a membraneous stomatitis. In addition there is a marked predisposition to both acute pericoronitis and acute ulcerative gingivitis.

The gingivostomatitis may be the first sign of the disease with red swollen gingivae which bleed easily and are similar to the gingival condition found in acute leukaemia or scurvy. Acute ulcerative gingivitis may be later superimposed upon this gingivitis. In up to 40 per cent of the patients petechiae and red macules occur on the soft palate, which are quite specific and so of diagnostic importance in this disease. Membrane formation may occur in the mouth, usually in the lower third molar region, as it frequently does in the fauces. The age of the patients involved means that acute pericoronitis and infectious mononucleosis may occur together, but the association is probably greater than fortuitous. The role of upper respiratory tract (virus) infections in the aetiology of acute pericoronitis is well recognized. There is no specific treatment for infectious mononucleosis.

Serious complications are rare and the course of glandular fever is variable; some patients recover very quickly while in others the disease runs a protracted course with the patient feeling generally unwell for some months. Treatment is purely symptomatic.

Coxsackie Infections

Aetiology

The Coxsackie viruses are a subgroup of the small (20–30 μ) RNA-based picorna viruses. The Coxsackie group is subdivisible into groups A and B on the basis of lesions induced in suckling mice. There are 23 viruses in group A and 6 in group B which between them cause a spectrum of illness which includes 'poliomyelitis', pleurodynia, aseptic meningitis, encephalitis, myocarditis and minor febrile illnesses with or without a rash. The two oral diseases are herpangina and hand foot and mouth disease.

Herpangina: This was first described by Zahorsky in 1920 and is due to Coxsackie A 2, 4, 5, 6, 8, 10 and 22. It is a disease principally of children and characterized by a sudden onset with fever and sore throat. Examination reveals upper cervical lymphadenopathy and intra-orally typical lesions occur on the soft palate, occasionally extending to the mouth or pharynx. The lesions are minute vesicles which rapidly ulcerate, on an acutely inflamed base, and up to a dozen may be noted on the palate. The disease is self-limited and resolves within a week.

Hand Foot and Mouth Disease: This is an acute infection due to Coxsackie A 16 (or rarely A 5 or 9). A short incubation period of 2–5 days is succeeded by painful oral ulceration and rash on the hands and feet with a negligible systemic upset (except in infants). In mild cases only oral lesions may be present and they consist of small vesicles which break down to form ulcers indistinguishable from aphthae on an erythematous base. The skin lesions consist of little areas of erythema which rarely may vesiculate. The lesions remit in 10 days. The diagnosis may be proved by virus isolation or a rise in specific antibody titre.

Measles

Koplik's spots are the characteristic oral feature of this disease, named after the famous American paediatrician, Henry Koplik, who lived during the nineteenth and twentieth centuries. Contrary to popular belief, these spots do not occur at any specific time in the disease and may even appear after the rash. When they do occur early with catarrhal symptoms, diagnosis is possible before the rash appears. Koplik's spots appear on the buccal or labial mucosa and being small and numerous give the mucosa a granular appearance; surrounding mucosa appears red with the spots appearing white. Their presence is one of the marked differences between measles and rubella, which also lack catarrhal features, but may be associated with suboccipital lymphadenopathy.

Virally-induced Epithelial Hyperplasias

   a. Poxviruses
      i. Molluscum contagiosum.
   b. Papovaviruses
      i. Verrucae.
      ii. Condyloma acuminatum.
      iii. Focal epithelial hyperplasia.
   c. ? Agent
      i. Keratoacanthoma.

Molluscum Contagiosum: This is due to a brick-shaped DNA-based poxvirus and has been reported on the lips and very rarely on oral mucosa. The lesions grow rapidly but after 2 months or so regress. Being unusual in the mouth they are not diagnosed until excised for biopsy.

Verrucae: The papovaviruses are associated with a number of epithelial responses which are clinically distinct. Why this should be so is not clear but may be related to different strains of virus and genetic factors in the host.

Common warts (verrucae vulgaris) are the common manifestation which are more common in children, are obviously infective, and tend to spontaneous cure. Warts do occur in the mouth where they are clinically and pathologically indistinguishable from papillomas. Warts are considered likely if the lesion occurs in childhood (especially if lesions are present on the skin and in the anterior part of the mouth).

Condyloma Acuminatum: This is a sessile genital wart from which infection is transferred to the oral cavity; oral lesions rather like broadly based less papilliferous warts result. The surface (as in warts) is white. Again the lesion is essentially undiagnosable due to its rarity and may be recognized retrospectively from the histology after excision. Most are probably diagnosed as papillomata (which they are).

Focal (Oral) Epithelial Hyperplasia (Heck's Disease): This is an oral mucosal abnormality occurring almost exclusively among Eskimos and American Indians. In the Americas the general prevalence is less than 3·5 per cent while in Greenland the general level is 7 per cent with pockets as high as 36 per cent.

The histological features include acanthosis and increased cellularity of the epithelium with some enlarged cells with ballooned and degenerate nuclei. These cells are filled with virus particles.

Clinical features

Among American Indians lesions are common in children while in Eskimos they are most frequent in middle-age. Lesions occur on the lower lip, cheeks and on the tongue. They are slightly raised light pink soft nodules which are well circumscribed and usually multiple. They are symptomless.

Keratoacanthoma: This bears all the hallmarks of a virally-induced epithelial hyperplasia but there is no proof of a viral aetiology.

Pathologically the lesion bears a close resemblance to squamous-cell carcinoma (the clinical resemblance is also close) due to the extreme epithelial hyperplasia. If the lesion has been excised whole, however, it can be usually recognized by the pathologist.

Clinically the lesions occur on the skin including the vermilion border of the lips and *exceptionally* intraorally. They present rapidly enlarging intracutaneous nodules with a pearly lobulated surface and a central crater. The maximum size is 2 cm and that is normally achieved within

3 months when spontaneous involution is the rule. They are remarkably like carcinomas and in case of doubtful nature excision is to be preferred to observation.

Bibliography

Archard H. O., Heck J. W. and Stanley H. R. (1965) An unusual oral mucosal lesion found in Indian children. *Oral Surg.* **20**, 201.

Banks P. (1967) Infectious mononucleosis. *Br. J. Oral Surg.* **4**, 227.

Burnett G. W. and Scherp H. W. (1976) *Oral Microbiology and infectious disease.* 4th ed. Baltimore, Williams & Wilkins.

Cawson R. A. and McSwiggan D. A. (1969) An outbreak of hand-foot and mouth disease in a dental hospital. *Oral Surg.* **27**, 451.

Farmer E. D. (1956) Diseases of the mouth caused by the *herpes simplex* virus. *Proc. R. Soc. Med.* **49**, 640.

Forman L. and Whitwell G. P. B. (1934) The association of *herpes catarrhalis* with erythema multiforme (Hebra). *Br. J. Dermatol.* **46**, 309.

Fraser-Moodie W. A. (1967) The oral lesions in infectious mononucleosis. *Oral Surg.* **12**, 685.

Lehner T. et al. (1975) Immunological basis for latency, recurrences and putative oncogenicity of herpes simplex virus. *Lancet,* **2**, 60.

Niederman J. C., McCollum R. W., Henle G. and Henle W. (1968) Infectious mononucleosis: clinical manifestations in relation to EB virus antibodies. *JAMA* **203**, 205.

Praetorius-Clausen F. (1972) Rare oral viral disorders (molluscum contagiosum, verrucae, condyloma accuminatum and focal epithelial hyperplasia. *Oral Surg.* **34**, 604.

Praetorius-Clausen F., Mongeltoft M., Roed-Peterson B. and Pindborg J. J. (1970) Focal epithelial hyperplasia of the oral mucosa in a South-west Greenlandic population. *Scand. J. Dent. Res.* **78**, 287.

Schiff B. L. (1958) Molluscum contagiosum of the buccal mucosa. *Arch. Dermatol.* **78**, 90.

Southam J. L. (1969) Recurrent intra-oral *Herpes simplex* infection. *Br. Dent. J.* **127**, 276.

Southam J. L., Colley I. T. and Clarke N. G. (1968) Oral herpetic infection in adults. *Br. J. Dermatol.* **80**, 248.

Chapter 4

Oral Infections (Bacterial and Fungal)

In this chapter will be considered the suppurative infections around the jaws which originate in dental diseases and also the specific infections, namely:

1. Actinomycosis.
2. Fusospirochaetal infections.
3. Candidosis.
4. Tuberculosis.
5. Syphilis.
6. Whooping cough.
7. Scarlet fever.
8. Diphtheria.
9. Tetanus.
10. Miscellaneous infestations.

Suppurative Infections

Around the jaws almost all acute suppurative infections originate in the teeth—the few that do not are due to skin sepsis. As these dental infections are themselves consequent upon the ravages of dental caries or periodontal disease or are associated with pericoronitis a few words about these is not out of place.

Dental Caries: This is due to the metabolism of sugars by oral bacteria with the production of acid which causes decalcification of the tooth substance. Central to the problem is the localization of the bacteria, substrate and acid on the tooth which is probably a function of the dental plaque. Plaque consists of dextrans which are polymerized by oral bacteria and mucopolysaccharides derived from the saliva. The bacteria implicated in acid production have been lactobacilli but lately attention has been focused more and more on streptococci (although this may be a nosological rather than an actual change). Factors in the aetiology of dental caries may be considered under three headings:

1. The resistance of the tooth.
2. The control of the plaque.
3. The soluble environment of the tooth: basically, the diet and saliva.

1. The tooth is weakened at sites of natural faults—enamel fissures and pits or lamellae or in areas of pathological calcification (enamel hypoplasia).

Trace elements in the enamel are important in its resistance, fluorine being the most important, best taken by ingestion in the drinking water during the time of tooth formation but topically applied fluoride has a limited effectiveness also.

2. Plaque formation is influenced by the diet, both by its chemical constituents and physical nature. The modern glutinous diet which almost completely lacks an abrasive or detergent action demands, in substitution, efficient oral hygiene.

3. The modern diet's high content of glucose and disaccharides which may be rapidly transformed into plaque dextrans or catabolized to acid is disastrous to the teeth, particularly with the modern habit of constant chewing of sugary foods. Sucrose particularly is as dangerous a foodstuff as a recently banned substitute (cyclamates) but cariogenicity does not carry the same notoriety as (potential) carcinogenicity. Dental caries destroys the crown of the tooth, which is endowed with only feeble defensive reactions. When the caries exposes the pulp chamber oral bacteria colonize the pulp chamber, frequently without symptoms although acute pulpitis may occur. The pulp is destroyed and the bacteria excite an inflammatory response in the periapical tissues which may be acute but is more usually chronic. Such a non-vital tooth would be exfoliated but for its layer of cementum which remains vital, protected from bacteria and their products in the pulp and dentinal tubules by the impermeable primary cementum. The chronic periapical granuloma may contain an abscess cavity and the epithelium of the rests of Malassez may be stimulated to form a periapical (*syn.* radicular or dental) cyst. The cyst, once formed, enlarges spontaneously and is no longer dependent upon the infective process for its persistence. At any point ingress of virulent bacteria into a chronically infected pulp chamber may lead to acute infection.

Periodontal Disease: This is again due to the effect of oral bacteria in dental plaque causing inflammation in gingival tissue The basic cause is the lack of a detergent diet which scours plaque off teeth and gums. The development of periodontal disease is more closely related to lack of oral hygiene, which acts as a substitute for the cleansing action of a proper diet, than is dental caries. Periodontal disease passes through the stages of chronic gingivitis and then periodontitis with loss of alveolar bone. Acute infection may punctuate the course of chronic periodontitis but is usually well localized as an acute paradontal abscess. On rare occasions lymphadenitis or tissue-space infection may originate in periodontal disease.

Pericoronitis: This is a bacterial infection of the tissues around the crown of a tooth and for practical purposes only occurs around the lower third molar although eruption of the upper wisdom is occasionally complicated by pericoronitis.

Acute pericoronitis is due to relatively virulent organisms and is predisposed by upper respiratory tract infections but the most important single feature in the aetiology is trauma to the pericoronal tissue by the corresponding upper third (or second) molar. Acute pericoronitis has a rapid onset with pain, swelling and trismus with malaise and fever. The swelling occurs within the mouth but also externally over and beneath the angle of the mandible. Tender submandibular lymphadenopathy is invariably associated. Acute pericoronitis may be difficult to distinguish from quinsy though in the latter dysphagia is more marked, external swelling is absent and the lymph nodes involved are upper deep cervical. Examination in the mouth in pericoronitis reveals inflammation around the wisdom tooth which may be invisible but is usually palpable and a bead of pus is present over the crown. The offending tooth may be demonstrated by extra-oral radiography. Treatment consists of antibiotics and hot salt mouth baths. If the upper wisdom is traumatizing the lower soft tissue it must be removed at the earliest opportunity. In the rare event of the associated wisdom tooth being in a normal eruptive path with room to fully erupt, it may be retained, but in the great majority of cases this not the case and the tooth should be removed under antibiotic cover as soon as the acute phase is past.

Chronic pericoronitis is a grumbling inflammatory process characterized by local tenderness and purulent discharge from around the crown of the partly erupted tooth. X-ray of the tooth shows solution of bone around the crown of the tooth. The offending wisdom tooth should again be removed as soon as possible under antibiotic cover. In some cases a subacute stage may be recognized with abscess formation and pus may track forward in the buccal sulcus to point well forward. Such a burrowing abscess often leads to diagnostic difficulties and first or second molars may be mistakenly removed before the diagnosis becomes clear.

From these primary sources of infection may be derived the dentoalvolar abscess which is a consequence of periapical infection and there may be involvement of local tissue spaces, suppurative lymphadenitis or osteomyelitis. In all such cases essentially the same bacteria are involved and the bacteriology will be considered. Also there is frequent reference to antibiotics and since the same therapy applies to all, that aspect of treatment will also be considered here to avoid repetition.

Bacteriology

These dental infections are frequently mixed but in the majority of cases streptococci are the principal organisms isolated. These may be α or γ-streptococci and a high percentage are anaerobes. β-haemolytic streptococci are recovered infrequently. Staphylococci may occur from time to time (10 per cent)—usually coagulase negative strains and micrococci occur in equally small numbers. Among the bacilli, either diphtheroids or lactobacilli may be present, but the most frequently isolated are various enterobacilli—particularly *Escherichia*. Yeasts are not infrequently isolated. In such mixed infections there seems little doubt that many organisms are passengers and the streptococci are the principal invaders.

Antibiotic therapy

The part played by streptococci in dental infections is underlined by the unquestioned value of penicillin in their treatment. For an 'average' case oral therapy is adequate; after a loading dose of 500 mg phenoxymethyl penicillin the treatment is continued at 250 mg qds. The dose may be maintained at 500 mg qds if the infection is more severe. For severe infections parenteral therapy is essential and to be practical this demands admission to hospital. Crystalline penicillin is then given in a dose of 1 million units bd intramuscularly and in the most severe cases the frequency of such injections may be doubled. Although such a regime provides only intermittent high therapeutic blood levels of penicillin, it proves quite satisfactory in practice. It is preferred by some to use 500 000 IU of crystalline penicillin with 300 000 IU of procaine penicillin intramuscularly bd which provides more prolonged although low blood levels. If the patient is allergic to penicillin either erythromycin or tetracycline may be employed (both at 250 mg qds after a loading dose of 500 mg), but tetracycline is to be avoided in children below 10 years.

Either is suitable as a second choice for an infection which fails to respond to penicillin but in such a case the choice of an alternative antibiotic should depend on the results of sensitivity tests which become available after 48 hours. There is very rarely a need to use antibiotics other than these three, but in special cases lincomycin or ampicillin may be indicated. Metronidazole 200 mg tds is an effective substitute for penicillin in the treatment of acute dental infections.

Dento-alveolar Abscess

Aetiology and pathology

This, as noted above, derives from acute periapical infection which is most commonly a sequel to exposure of the pulp by dental caries. On occasion a vital pulp may be infected from a high lateral root canal or via lymphatics when there is associated periodontal pocketing. A tooth rendered non-vital by trauma, or by chemical or physical insults to the coronal dentine as in conservation, may become infected either by periodontal lymphatics or during the course of a bacteraemia. Exposure of the pulp due to trauma also inevitably leads to periapical infection unless rapidly treated.

In an acute infection due to virulent bacteria suppuration develops at the apex of the tooth and the subsequent direction taken by the pus is governed by anatomical factors, firstly the relationship of the apex to the cortical bony plate of the jaw and secondly, once in the soft tissues, the muscle and fascial attachments around the jaws.

Pus from upper cheek teeth usually penetrates the thin buccal plate below the origin of the buccinator and so points within the buccal sulcus in the mouth. On occasion pus from an upper canine or upper first molar extends above the buccinator origin to present in the cheek. From the upper incisor region pus may exceptionally extend into the nose but usually presents within the labial vestibule. The lateral incisor apex and that of the palatal root of the first molar are close to the palatal surface of the maxilla and so may give rise to a palatal abscess, which, if left untreated, points at the junction of the hard and soft palates.

Likewise, from the lower teeth pus tracks most commonly to the buccal side except from the third or second molars, of which the apices lie closer to the lingual side and the pus emerges below the mylohyoid muscle to present in the submandibular space and points in the neck. From the remaining lower teeth the pus presents buccally in the vestibule although that from a first molar may be below buccinator origin and so present on the facial skin. Abscesses of lower incisors may present on the point of the chin the pus being guided by the mentalis muscle.

Clinical features

The dento-alveolar abscess may be acute or chronic. In the most acute case there is an explosive onset, usually with no premonitory symptoms referable to the teeth. There is a rapidly developing, throbbingly painful swelling. From the upper anterior teeth the swelling may extend with closure of the eye due to periorbital oedema. The central area of the swelling over the teeth is tender, indurated and overlying skin may be red, but the majority of the swelling is not tender and represents inflammatory oedema and not cellulitis as it is frequently termed. Examination in the buccal sulcus reveals a tender swelling which obliterates the depths of the vestibule and inflammation extends down to the attached mucosa. The point at which infection tracks from the apex of the offending tooth is more readily felt than seen. With the onset of suppuration, in 2–3 days the swelling tends to localize with absorption of the circumferential oedema and towards the end of the first week the abscess points at the site indicated above.

In many cases this very acute onset is lacking and the condition is less dramatic without the peripheral oedema, and in such cases more pus is formed and marked fluctuation is common.

There is always regional (submandibular) lymphadenopathy and although the patient may have a slight fever he shows few, if any, signs of the systemic upset associated with infective disease and any general symptoms are more related to pain and sleeplessness than to 'toxaemia'. The blood shows mild neutrophil leucocytosis and the ESR is temporarily raised. A chronic dental abscess is unusual in adults and is usually due to antibiotic treatment leaving the basic cause—the tooth—untreated. Abscesses of the deciduous teeth are commonly chronic and well localized to the associated alveolus and such has been termed a parulis.

A discharging sinus always remains if a dento-alveolar abscess is left untreated or is treated improperly and may also develop silently from chronic periapical infection. On occasion the mouth of a sinus develops exuberant granulations which may closely resemble a pyogenic granuloma. External sinuses develop most frequently as noted above in connection with lower incisors (the median mental sinus) and first molars, especially the lower. In such cases the presence of a dense fibrotic band joining the skin to the underlying jaw is obvious.

The tooth which is the origin of the abscess may be immediately obvious, being either visibly non-vital with a greyish discoloration or grossly carious or heavily filled. The tooth is very tender to touch (periostitic) but adjacent teeth may be similarly tender. Radiographic examination may be necessary to distinguish the offending tooth which is revealed by a periapical radiolucency, but this is by no means invariable.

Treatment

In the first instance the causative tooth has to be extracted or root-filled so that the focus of infection in the pulp chamber is eliminated. Root filling may be undertaken in any tooth but is usually limited to those with a single root, the upper incisors and canines and lower incisors, canines and premolars. The tooth must also have a crown subsequently capable of restoration, a root with no anatomical abnormality and a sound periodontal condition. Patients over 60 years are generally unsuitable for root-canal therapy as are most patients with a cardiac condition predisposing to infective endocarditis. The overriding influence is the willingness of the patient to undertake treatment which involves multiple visits. If root treatment is to be performed the tooth should be widely opened to drain the root canal and for this general anaesthesia may be required but the airotor has rendered the procedure relatively painless in its absence. A course of antibiotics may be indicated and when the acute phase is past the root-canal treatment is completed. In the majority of cases extraction under general anaesthesia is the only treatment required but with an extensive soft-tissue abscess incision may also be indicated. Antibiotics are only indicated in the severe cases, if the patient has a cardiac condition predisposing to subacute bacterial endocarditis, is a diabetic or on steroids or has some disorder lowering systemic resistance. Antibiotic therapy may be used as a primary treatment if definitive measures have to be delayed. This is justified if the patient has a haemorrhagic diathesis or is unfit for a general anaesthetic but is frequently undertaken if facilities for general anaesthesia are not available and the tooth may be subsequently removed under local analgesia.

Following extraction during the acute phase the swelling may increase slightly but remits during the succeeding week. On occasion the soft-tissue infection persists following extraction and a loculus of pus forms and then incision and antibiotic therapy are required.

Subperiosteal Osteomyelitis: In some cases an acute dental abscess strips up the periosteum and there follows cortical sequestration or solution with some surrounding bone production which condition has been termed subperiosteal osteomyelitis. The condition is not infrequently associated with the submasseteric abscess, considered elsewhere. In such cases surgical exploration and prolonged antibiotic therapy is desirable.

Alveolar Abscess in the Edentulous: An alveolar abscess in the edentulous or in an edentulous area of the jaws demands radiography to reveal the underlying cause, which is a buried tooth or root or a dental cyst. On occasion no such cause can be discovered and in these cases it is probable that the infection is due to foreign material being forced through the soft tissues by the denture.

Infected Dental Cyst: This is clincially indistinguishable from a dentoalveolar abscess but radiography immediately reveals the true state of affairs.

Tissue Space Infections

These may arise from pericoronal or periapical (rarely periodontal) infection but on occasion are due to a dirty needle and may follow extraction of teeth. These 'spaces' are potential rather than actual and are areas of soft tissue bounded by bone, muscle and deep fascia which are resistant to transgression by invading organisms. Consideration will be given to infections of the:

1. Submandibular space.
2. Sublingual space.
3. Lateral pharyngeal space.
4. Submasseteric space.
and
5. Ludwig's angina (a combined infection).
6. Acute suppurative lymphadenitis.

1. **Submandibular Space:** This may be infected from the apices of the lower second and third molars or from the enclosed salivary or lymph glands. It is characterized by swelling in the submandibular region with some swelling in the floor of the mouth and the patient feels unwell and has a fever. The swelling is brawny and tender and the overlying skin inflamed.

   In all such acute infections about the jaws considerable difficulty may be experienced in distinguishing those in which suppuration has occurred and would thus benefit from incision and drainage. The initial treatment should be with antibiotics but if the condition deteriorates or does not improve in 48 hours incision is indicated.

2. **Sublingual Space:** The space, which is bilateral, lies above the mylohyoid muscle and may be infected from the apices of the lower premolars, canines and incisors, following extraction or by needle track infection. Swelling due to the laxity of the tissues is extreme but principally intra-oral, the tongue being pushed upward and the floor of the mouth elevated to obliterate the lingual sulcus. Submental swelling is less prominent. This is treated as for the submandibular space infection but incision, if called for, is performed intra-orally.

3. **Lateral Pharyngeal Space:** This lies between the medial pterygoid and the superior constrictor muscles and is infected by extension of acute pericoronitis. In the majority of cases of distal spread of infection from the wisdom tooth, the lateral limit is the superior constrictor and the infection tracks upward beneath the mucosa to present clinically as a paratonsillar abscess (quinsy). In such a case there is external swelling and submandibular lymphadenitis due to the original pericoronitis but symptomatically distinguished by very painful dysphagia in addition to extreme trismus. Intra-oral examination reveals the features of acute pericoronitis with, in addition, gross swelling of the anterior pillar of the fauces and ipsilateral soft palate with maximum swelling at the upper pole of the tonsil.

Treatment is, in the first instance, with antibiotics but in the absence of rapid improvement incision is required; however *great care* is required during the *induction of anaethesia*. Acute infections lateral to the superior constrictor but medial to the ascending ramus are usually due to needle track infection following inferior dental nerve block and are associated with persistent anaesthesia of the lip, pain and trismus. They are successfully treated with antibiotics.

4. **Submasseteric Space:** This lies between the masseter and the ascending ramus of the jaw and infection spreads from the lower wisdom tooth either following pericoronitis or removal of the tooth. There is extensive tender swelling over the ascending ramus with complete trismus; if the infection is at all prolonged subperiosteal osteomyelitis of the ascending ramus is not infrequent. The collection of pus may be aspirated but operation is often required to release it and again great care is required with induction of anaesthesia. Antibiotics are again indicated as soon as the condition is diagnosed.

5. **Ludwig's Angina:** This very rare infection is a combination of sub-lingual and bilateral submandibular space involvement with spread down the neck and laryngeal oedema, hence stridor and dysphagia. It demands immediate very high antibiotic dosage, surgical incision to relieve tension and maintenance of fluid and nutritional balance by intravenous or intragastric drip.

6. **Acute Suppurative Lymphadenitis:** Tender regional lymphadenitis is invariably associated with suppurative dental infections (except actinomycosis) but on occasion the lymphadenitis assumes greater importance than the primary source of infection with severe inflammation and suppuration. Such acute severe lymphadenitis in the submandibular region is commonly associated with a relatively inconspicuous primary (dental) source but rarely complicates severe infections such as dento-alveolar abscess or acute pericoronitis. It may also follow cutaneous, nasal or pharyngeal (including tonsillar or ear) infection while on occasion no primary source can be discovered. This condition is more common in children and particularly those of Negro extraction. In all cases there is sudden severe painful submandibular swelling which is associated with inflammation of the overlying skin. Palpation may reveal one or two very enlarged nodes but usually periadentis is too great and the nodes are impalpable. At this stage it is impossible to distinguish this condition from acute submandibular space infection and acute sialadenitis. Full clinical and radiological examination is essential to establish the primary source. Antibiotics are the treatment of choice with early incision for drainage if resolution does not occur. There is no need to eliminate the primary source of infection at this stage, unless convenient; it is best dealt with when the acute phase is past. There is a detailed consideration of cervical lymphadenopathy in Chapter 20.

Apart from these acute infections osteomyelitis of the jaws is for practical purposes due to infections of dental origin but is beyond the scope of this book.

Finally, such infections may spread by direct extension to the mediastinum or cavernous sinus or by the bloodstream to produce cerebral abscesses. Aspirated material from the mouth may lead to pulmonary abscesses.

Actinomycosis

This is a subacute or chronic infection due to actinomyces which occurs most frequently around the jaws and is closely related in its pathogenesis to dental infection and tooth extraction but on rare occasions occurs in the lungs and ileocaecal regions.

Aetiology and pathogenesis

Actinomyces israelii is the aetiological agent and it is a Gram-positive organism which shows true branching. The size is 12–15 × 2 μm but the hyphae tend to remain together to form matted colonies which are the 'sulphur-granules' in the pus and account for the name ray-fungus. The organism is anaerobic and may be cultured. Actinomycotic pus almost invariably also contains a large number of small Gram-negative bacilli which are identified as either *Actinobacillus actinomycetocomitans* or *Bacteroides corrodens* which are thought by some authorities to be important in the aetiology and persistence of the lesion. This view is largely untenable because although these organisms are resistant to penicillin and sometimes to tetracycline both these drugs are effective in the management of actinomycosis. They may play a part in the colonization of the tissues by rendering local conditions suitable for actinomyces. *Actinomyces israelii* can be recovered from the normal mouth. On the rare occasions when it invades the tissues it excites an intense neutrophil polymorph reaction. The infection spreads centrifugally with a strong tendency to erode through the skin. The regional lymph nodes are never enlarged in connection with an actinomycotic focus but may be involved by direct spread. In chronic cases extensive fibrosis follows with a branching abscess cavity with one or more sinuses. On rare occasions the cortical plate of the mandible is eroded with some sequestration reminiscent of that of dento-alveolar abscess with subperiosteal abscess. True osteomyelitis due to this organism does not occur. The organism has been isolated not infrequently from periapical granulomas.

Clinical features

The infection rarely gains ingress through a deep periodontal pocket or the pericoronal space but more frequently via a tooth so that a dento-alveolar abscess is first formed. The most usual mode of infection is, however, that which follows extraction of lower molars, the third molar in particular, and may complicate fractures through the angle of the mandible. Exceptionally, the disease may follow extraction of other mandibular teeth or the upper first molar. In all such post-extraction cases the symptoms usually develop 1–6 weeks later. In any event the onset may be acute, as a rapidly developing, painful swelling which is well localized, but on occasion is identical with the most severe dento-alveolar abscess with extensive surrounding oedema. The onset is usually less dramatic, even self-effacing; the patient notices a small swelling overlying the mandible or in the submandibular region which may be intermittent at first but is usually progressive. In all cases there is a strong tendency to involve the skin and in all but the most acute this gradually thins to form a bluish excresence over the centre of a swelling which is fluctuant. In all cases there is good clinical evidence for incision and drainage. If left untreated (which is quite exceptional nowadays) the skin breaks down with discharge and the lesion extends with progressive induration. Regional lymphadenopathy is characteristically absent as noted above.

Diagnosis is established by examination of the pus which, in suspicious cases, should be collected in a tube. Direct examination of the pus reveals the organism and its presence is confirmed by culture.

Treatment

The invariable need for incision (or aspiration) and the diagnostic value of that procedure is noted above. Subsequently, antibiotic treatment is required; either penicillin or tetracycline may be used. Most known strains are sensitive to penicillin but colonies of the organism are relatively resistant and since the organism frequently exists in the tissues in colonial form, high and prolonged dosage is required. Intramuscular penicillin is the ideal (600 000 IU procaine penicillin bd for 1 month followed for 1 month by 250 mg penicillin V tablets qds). This is a remarkably inconvenient schedule for an ambulant patient and tablets of penicillin V 500 mg qds may replace the procaine penicillin noted above. In patients allergic to penicillin, or simply on the grounds of convenience and the more regular absorption of oral tetracycline, this may be preferred in a dose of 250 mg qds for 1–2 months; in fact, it is regarded by many as the drug of choice. It has been suggested by Rud that sulphonamides should be given as well but there is no evidence to support this assertion.

Fusospirochaetal Infections

Acute Ulcerative Gingivitis—Syn: Vincent's gingivitis, trench mouth, acute necrotizing ulcerative gingivitis: This is an acute ulcerative disorder probably due to fusospirochaetal infection, which usually affects the gingival margin but is occasionally more extensive. The other fusospirachaetal infections of the mouth include Vincent's angina and cancrum oris. Jean Hyacinthe Vincent, the French bacteriologist, described fusospirochaetal tonsillitis in 1898.

Aetiology

Swabs from the lesions always show a predominance of two organisms, namely a spirochaete, *Treponema vincentii*, and the cigarshaped *Fusiformis fusiformis*.

Treponema vincentii is the name for a group of organisms of variable morphology. Each organism consists of a loose outer membrane which encloses a spiral cytoplasmic cylinder wound around a bunch of axial filaments (rather like a caduceus) with an overall size of 8–12 × 0·5 μm. The organism is sensitive to penicillin and metronidazole but quantitative assessment is impossible. *Fusiformis fusiformis* is a cigar-shaped organism which is Gram-negative, either small 2–3 μ or large 6–8 μ × 0·75 μm. It is a facultative anaerobe and is highly sensitive to penicillin, other antibiotics and metronidazole.

The treponeme is non-pathogenic to mice, but the fusiforms may produce local infection in these animals. The two together are quite pathogenic in experimental animals but an explanation for this is not forthcoming. The presence of these bacteria in the lesion of Vincent's gingivitis suggests an aetiological relationship but the disease is communicable by the closest personal contact with difficulty.

Further evidence for their importance is the rapid resolution with penicillin or metronidazole with a parallel alteration in the bacterial flora of the lesions. The organisms are, however, normal oral inhabitants and very important to the aetiology of this infection are two predisposing factors.

Pre-existing gingivitis is the most important single factor and its cause is poor oral hygiene. The teeth are commonly stained, calculus is much in evidence and materia alba; irregularity and crowding of the teeth, which lead to stagnation areas, are common. Cigarette smoking is thought to be an important factor and may operate by reducing gingival blood supply. The only other local factor is the erupting wisdom tooth around which the pericoronal space forms a focus of stagnation which may lead to infection.

Systemic factors include many which frequently occur together so that the relative importance of each cannot be assessed. These factors are overwork, disturbed nights, anxiety, exposure to cold or damp, upper respiratory infections and undue exertion. Any, or all, of these factors account for the high incidence in servicemen and for 'epidemics' which occurred in the First World War of 'trench mouth'. In summary, the disease is an endogenous infection in which predisposing factors play a major role.

Pathology

Histopathology of the ulcer shows a surface pseudomembrane of fibrin, polymorphs, organisms (fusospirochaetal) and epithelial cells. This is covered by an ordinary bacterial plaque and materia alba. The actual surface of the ulcer teems with fusospirochaetal organisms and the adjacent tissue (the floor of the ulcer and the epithelium at the edge of the ulcer) is penetrated to a depth of about 300 µm by the spirochaetes. The tissue of the floor of the ulcer shows acute inflammation.

Incidence

The disease is more common in men than women, is most unusual before puberty with a peak incidence at 20–25 years. It is much more common in the autumn and winter, diminishing in the spring and especially the summer. It is rare in the tropics (but, as will be noted later, acute ulcerative gingivitis is not unusual among Nigerian infants).

Clinical features

The major symptoms are bleeding gums, soreness of the mouth, a bad taste or bad breath. On occasion, pain may occur but only in a case superimposed upon advanced periodontal disease with deep pocketing. Examination reveals the typical gingival ulceration which starts in the interdental area but is first observed on the interdental papilla. The ulceration spreads around the gingival margin of the adjacent teeth but is always more marked around the labial or buccal side than on the lingual or palatal. The disease often appears to involve several adjacent papillae simultaneously and the lower incisor region is that most frequently involved. The gingiva of a few teeth, or the whole mouth, may be involved.

The ulcers are narrow, up to 2 mm wide, and covered with an off-white slough which, if removed, reveals the concave bleeding floor. The margin of the ulcer is clear cut as if with a knife and the adjacent attached gingiva is acutely inflamed. On occasion, the ulceration extends over the attached gingiva rather than around the free gingival margin so that quite an extensive local ulcer may be formed. Rarely, contact ulcers may form on the side of tongue or on the cheek. Regional lymphadenopathy may occur but fever and systemic disturbance are exceptional although the patient may complain of feeling 'under the weather'. Halitosis is marked and some observers can recognize the disease by its characteristic smell. Vincent's gingivitis may complicate such disorders as acute leukaemia, cytotoxic drug therapy, agranulocytosis or infectious mononucleosis. If the patient complains of systemic upset these should be excluded by haematological examination.

Treatment

This should be both local and systemic. Systemic treatment consists of either penicillin or metronidazole—the latter being the drug of choice. Metronidazole is given in tablets of 200 mg tds for one week. Penicillin, if used, is conveniently given as phenoxymethyl penicillin 250 mg qds for one week. Pain is controlled in less than 12 hours and bleeding in less than 24 hours and the ulcers heal within 3–4 days. Local treatment consists initially of superficial scaling and the patient should be instructed to clean the teeth gently with a soft brush. Frequent mouth washes with diluted hydrogen peroxide are an aid to oral hygiene.

At the subsequent visit the teeth should be scaled and polished and arrangements made for necessary conservation, periodontal treatment and extractions, and oral hygiene instruction is given. Due to the destruction of the papillae, food traps are produced which are a source of chronic gingivitis so that gingivoplasty should be considered in each case. Unfortunately, many patients who develop the infection take no great care of their teeth and so suffer recurrences of the disease or the acute phase merges into chronic periodontal disease in which fusospirochaetal organisms undoubtedly play a part.

Vincent's Angina: This is an acute tonsillitis and pharyngitis due to the same organisms. The onset is acute with sore throat, malaise and cervical lymphadenopathy. Examination reveals single or multiple ulcers of the tonsils with a white pseudomembrane. It is to be distinguished from diphtheria by bacteriological examination and from infectious monucleosis by haematological investigation. In cases of doubt the patient should be treated as for diphtheria.

Cancrum Oris—Syn. Noma, Phagadena: This disease is now virtually confined to the tropics and appears to be due to fusospirochaetal infection in seriously debilitated infants and children and is characterized by rapidly progressive necrosis of the soft tissues about the jaws. It may occur in seriously ill adults such as the occupants of concentration camps where malnutrition and typhus appear to be important in the aetiology.

Aetiology and pathogenesis

Limited pathological studies indicate that the condition is identical to acute ulcerative gingivitis on a larger scale. The spirochaetes invade the vital tissue at the edge of the necrotic area and fusospirochaetal organisms cover the ulcerated surface. In the children studied by Emslie the disease appears to have originated as an acute ulcerative gingivitis which spread over adjacent soft tissue to expose alveolar bone and then extended into the lips, cheeks or tongue. Predisposing factors are a background of severe nutritional deficiency (but before the development of frank kwashiorkor) with anaemia due to hookworm infestation or malaria. On top of this are acute predisposition due to infection with either measles, smallpox or primary herpes infection (gingivostomatitis). The noma occurs during the later stages of measles and smallpox but follows the herpetic infection by a week or two.

Clinical features

The disease occurs in children with a maximum incidence at 3 years and the earliest stage is an often unrecognized acute ulcerative gingivitis. As spread occurs, induration develops and then necrosis as evidenced by a spreading black area in the skin. The ulceration and necrosis are progressive and a fatal outcome due to exhaustion and bronchopneumonia occurs in 90 per cent of untreated cases.

Treatment consists of penicillin and metronidazole and the treatment of all the underlying factors described above. Protein supplements are given with vitamins and iron and treatment for hookworm and malaria instituted as indicated.

Healing is by secondary intention with considerable fibrosis and consequent contraction of the defect. Severe extra-articular ankylosis of the temporomandibular joint is produced and early plastic surgery is necessary.

In parenthesis it is interesting to note that the diseases of the mouth and vagina are almost identical as are the reactions of their mucosae to hormonal cycles. The difference between the two is the absence of a fusospirochaetal vaginitis to correspond to acute ulcerative gingivitis (although noma occurs at each site) and trichomonal vaginitis which has no oral counterpart. Strange then that these two apparently dissimilar diseases, acute ulcerative gingivitis and trichomonal vaginitis are specifically treated with metronidazole!

Candidosis (*Syn*. Thrush, Moniliasis, Candidiasis)

An infection due to the yeast *Candida albicans* which, in the mouth, invades the superficial layers of epidermis only and has four distinct clinical expressions.

Aetiology and pathogenesis

The organism is a single-celled yeast of the family *Cryptococcaceae* which exists in one of three forms. The vegetative form is of yeast cells (blastospores) about 1·5–5 μm in diameter and oval in shape; a hyphal form of elongated cells is seen and chlamydospores which consist of cell bodies enclosed in a thick refractile wall with an overall diameter of 7–17 μm. The vegetative form is commonly the one found in the mouth, but if hyphae are present it is likely that the yeasts have direct aetiological relationship with any associated lesion.

The organism is resistant to cold but succumbs to heat of 50–60°C and is sensitive to aniline dyes such as methyl violet and brilliant green. Selective media include a peptone, maltose agar or broth at pH 5·0–5·5 (Sabouraud's medium) or a rice infusion or Tween 80 agar may be used. Anaerobic conditions are required for growth. The organisms may be found in up to 50 per cent of healthy mouths and about one-third of adult vaginae but is not normally found on the skin. Its persistence in the mouth and vagina is in part accounted for by a symbiotic relationship with *Lactobacillus acidophilus*, which organisms appear to favour persistence of the yeast, but by acid production limit its proliferation.

Candida albicans is of poor pathegenicity and infection demands predisposing factors which may be systemic or local. The systemic factors have been recognized for a century—in the words of Trousseau (1869) 'thrush is the local expression of a very bad state of the whole system' or Parrott (1877) 'thrush is always the result of predisposing malady' (Winner and Hurley, 1964). The predisposing factors are:

1. Infancy.
2. Endocrine disturbances
   a. Diabetes mellitus.
   b. Hypoparathyroidism.
   c. Hypoadrenalism.
   d. Steroid therapy.

    e. Pregnancy.
3. Malnutrition and malabsorption.
4. Severe blood dyscrasias.
5. Terminal malignant disease.
6. Postoperative debility.
7. Antibiotic treatment.

The local factors (on the skin) include chronic trauma to epithelium and intertrigenous areas or local skin disease with maceration.

Sources of infection

The normal vagina harbours *Candida albicans* in 10–15 per cent of adults and this figure doubles towards the end of pregnancy. As noted, pregnancy predisposes to vulvovaginitis but clinical infection occurs in only a fraction of these pregnant carriers. Children born of vaginal carriers acquire the yeasts at birth (and Lactobacilli) and are thirty-five times more likely to develop thrush than infants born to non-carriers, but only a small percentage of neonates (1 per cent) develop clinical thrush. Secondary spread to non-colonized neonates may take place in nurseries by human vector or feeding bottles. The neonates with the organism may develop clinical infection of the damp macerated skin of the nappy area. The neonatal skin is rapidly cleared of the organism and cutaneous candidosis occurs in premature babies or those with infantile eczema. Oral carriage persists in up to 50 per cent of adults, as noted above, and small numbers of the yeast are excreted in the faeces of one-third of these. In such a patient given antibiotics, large numbers of the organism are recoverable from the faeces and from an equal number without previous stool carriage. The organism colonizes the vagina after puberty, presumably from the anus, and the cycle is repeated to the next generation.

Pathology

Infection due to *Candida albicans* is usually superficial in the outer epidermis of the mouth, vagina and more rarely on the (abnormal) skin; only in severely debilitated persons does pulmonary or systemic infection occur. Acute infections excite little inflammatory response although interstitial collections of polymorphs (micro-abscesses) collect around the organisms. Superficial shedding of parakeratinized surface cells is usual. In chronic infections extreme epidermal hyperplasia may occur with hyperkeratosis, acanthosis and underlying chronic inflammatory cell infiltrate. The diagnosis of infection may prove difficult; the mere presence of the organism is not sufficient. Serological methods are not of any great help at the moment although Lehner has developed an immunofluorescent technique to quantitate serum and salivary antibodies. Histological demonstration of the organism within epithelium is diagnostic, using a PAS stain. Demonstration of hyphal forms and chlamydospores in a scraping from the lesion is conclusive and finally healing of the lesion with antifungal treatment may be a pointer.

Clinical features

The oral manifestations will be considered as follows (after Lehner):
  1. Acute
      a. Thrush (pseudomembranous candidosis).
      b. Atrophic candidosis (antibiotic stomatitis).
  2. Chronic
      a. Atrophic (denture sore mouth).
      b. Hyperplastic (candida leucoplakia).
  3. Chronic mucocutaneous candidosis.

1*a. Thrush:* Acute pseudomembranous candidosis. This is by far the commonest form of candidosis occuring in neonates and the severely debilitated. In neonates it is seen on the second to fifth day of life and presents as white curdy patches on the cheeks, lips, palate and tongue. The surrounding mucosa is not inflamed and the pseudomembrane may be removed with difficulty; a partly eroded area of oral mucosa is revealed. Spread may occur to the pharynx and oesophagus with feeding difficulty, regurgitation and weight loss. Among adults thrush occurs in debilitated patients with such disorders as disseminated malignancy, operations or treatment with antimitotics, steroids or antibiotics and combinations of these are frequent. Treatment of thrush in infants is readily effected by Nystatin suspension 1 ml (100 000 IU) four times daily. In adult cases attention to the underlying disorder is called for and local treatment consists of Nystatin tablets (500 000 IU) to be sucked four times daily. A suitable alternative to the rather unpleasant Nystatin is Amphotericin B 10 mg tablets used in the same way.

1*b. Acute atrophic candidosis:* This is simply thrush without the pseudomembrane and occurs particularly in association with antibiotic treatment and was formerly called antibiotic stomatitis or glossitis.

Examination reveals erosions of the oral mucosa which are sore and the dorsum of the tongue shows a characteristic patchy depapillation with the surrounding tongue thickly coated. It is treated as for thrush (*see above*).

2*a*. *Chronic atrophic candidosis. Syn.* Denture sore mouth, denture stomatitis: This condition, the commonest expression of oral candidosis, was first described by Cahn in 1936 and is due to *Candida* infection in an oral mucosa conditioned by a covering prosthesis. The area involved is usually the palate beneath partial or complete upper dentures; it is much less common beneath lower partial dentures and exceptional beneath the full lower denture. The condition is more common in women than men, occurring in one-quarter of female denture wearers but only one-tenth of the corresponding group of males. The important factors as far as the dentures are concerned are thought to be trauma and failure to leave the dentures out at night. Trauma is increased by poor fit, improper occlusal relationship and roughness of the fitting surface (possibly predisposed by an alginate impression). Important systemic predisposing factors are diabetes, anaemia and steroid therapy. Although the lesion may be patchy it usually involves the whole fitting surface beneath the upper denture up to the crest of the ridge but rarely extends over the labial or buccal side of the alveolus. The mucosa is bright red and has a pebbly surface as if the whole is covered by discrete but almost confluent blebs of 1–2 mm diameter. In the clefts between these blebs whitish fluid is present and patches of thrush may be noted. *Candida albicans* may be recovered from over 90 per cent of such palates. Further extension of the infection may take place on to the intertrigenous area of skin at the commissure of the lips and patients with angular cheilitis almost invariably have denture stomatitis (although only a small percentage of patients with denture stomatitis develop angular cheilitis). Its development depends upon the presence of a fold at the corner of the mouth which may be due to senile loss of skin electricity or denture faults such as overclosure or incorrect positioning of teeth. This leads to a triangle of skin bathed in saliva which is colonized by the yeasts. The appearances are of a small fissure running from the commissure surrounded by a pink or dull red area with a further surround of white macerated skin. It is sometimes associated with a triangular area of 'speckled' leucoplakia in a corresponding, though larger, area of the buccal mucosa adjacent to the commissure (*vide infra*). Vitamin-B deficiency plays no part in the aetiology of angular cheilitis as seen in this country.

Treatment of denture stomatitis is to leave out the offending denture and to prescribe Nystatin or Amphotericin B tablets as in thrush. In addition an expert prosthetic opinion is desirable to provide a sound basis for future prevention; new dentures are usually necessary. Many patients, however, refuse to leave out the denture during the day and the regime may be modified by relining the denture and correcting occlusal abnormalities. The denture should be left out for as long as possible and certainly at night when it should be soaked in 1 per cent cetrimide solution. During the day Nystatin suspension should be applied to the fitting surface of the upper denture three times daily. For additional angular cheilitis prosthetic replacement to eliminate the fold at the corner of the mouth is essential to a cure. Nystatin or Amphotericin B cream may be applied to the commissure to treat the lesion while the denture stomatitis is also treated as above. On rare occasions surgical treatment to eliminate the fold is necessary.

2b. *Chronic hyperplastic candidosis:* Candida leucoplakia: In this condition a white patch is present associated with extensive candidal infection in its epithelial layers but after elimination of the yeasts a patch of hyperplastic epithelium (leucoplakia) persists. Cawson, who originally defined the condition, considers the yeasts to be of primary importance in the aetiology of the epithelial hyperplasia.

The histopathology of this lesion differs from that of leucoplakia in that the epithelium is always parakeratinized and there is gross acanthosis which alternates with areas only a few cells thick. The superficial epithelium shows considerable intercellular oedema which separates the individual cells, and polymorphs infiltrate the epithelium. The deepest epithelial layers show intense proliferative activity with many mitoses and dyskeratosis is common. In Cawson's series among 128 non-dyskeratotic leucoplakias candidosis was present in 8 (6 per cent) while of 10 dyskeratotic lesions candidosis was present in 6 (60 per cent) or, put in another way, dyskeratosis is present in 40 per cent of cases of chronic hyperplastic candidosis but in only 3 per cent of leucoplakias. The same feature was noted by Jepsen and Winther who associated chronic candidosis with 'speckled' leucoplakia.

The underlying chorium shows intense chronic inflammatory cell infiltration and the lymphocytes may show an almost follicular arrangement. Using PAS stain *Candida* hyphae are demonstrable in the hyperplastic epithelium.

Clinically this form of candidosis is indistinguishable from leucoplakia although it has been particularly associated with speckled leucoplakia which occurs most frequently as a triangular patch inside the commissure of the lips bilaterally. Any site such as cheek, tongue or palate may be affected. Such a lesion may only be diagnosed on biopsy and occurs in adults with no apparent predisposition to *Candida* infection. This lesion is strongly precancerous, even when first seen there is often markedly dysplastic epithelium on biopsy, or even carcinoma. It is important to biopsy an erosive, red area to establish the 'worst' histological features. Such patients must be followed up very closely (3-monthly). These are the lesions for which a case can be made for excision and skin grafting.

Nystatin or Amphotericin B troches may be prescribed to be sucked four times daily but seem to have little effect.

There is a natural tendency to assume that the candidal infection plays an active role in the development of oral carcinoma at these sites, i.e. that the fungus itself is a carcinogenic agent. There is as yet no experimental demonstration of this and much clinical evidence speaks against it; particularly the non-occurrence of cancer in cases of chronic atrophic candidosis (a generally susceptible age group) and chronic mucocutaneous candidosis, admittedly not an age group in which oral cancer occurs but in some of which cancer is predisposed by the T-cell abnormalities.

Treatment is to use Nystatin tablets four times daily for several months but the infection is difficult to eradicate and, if it is a simple leucoplakia, persists. Carcinoma may supervene in such an area.

3. *Chronic mucocutaneous candidosis:* This is a rare group of disorders in which some systemic factor predisposes to extensive candidal infection of mucosae, nails and skin; of which oral involvement is usually a most important clinical feature. Classification of these cases is provisionally arranged as follows:

GROUP I

i. Familial multiple endocrinopathy and mucocutaneous candidosis (Higgs and Wells Group 3).

GROUP II: Primary T(thymic)-lymphocyte failure with diminished cellular immune response.

i. Swiss type agammaglobulinaemia (thymic aplasia).

ii. Di George syndrome—third and fourth branchial pouch dysplasia with thymic aplasia and absent parathyroid glands.

GROUP III

i. Familial chronic mucocutaneous candidosis (Higgs and Wells Group 1).

ii. Chronic mucocutaneous candidosis with granulomata and susceptibility to other infections (Higgs and Wells Group 2).

iii. Chronic mucocutaneous candidosis of late onset (Higgs and Wells Group 4).

GROUP I: *Familial multiple endocrinopathy and mucocutaneous candidosis* In this syndrome oral mucosal candidosis is usually the first clinical feature and generally develops before puberty, often in early childhood while the onset of endocrine disturbance follows several years later. In many cases there is chronic keratoconjunctivitis (another mucocutaneous ocular syndrome?). The commonest endocrine abnormality is hypoparathyroidism but hypoadrenocorticism, hypothyroidism, pernicious anaemia, chronic active hepatitis and Schilder's disease may also occur.

In this syndrome all these 'organ' failures appear to be due to allergic ('autoimmune') reactions. Multiple autoantibodies may be demonstrated. Possibly what is inherited is a defective 'suppressor' mechanism for forbidden clones.

GROUP II: In the group of patients with T-lymphocyte deficit and consequent failure to mount a cell-mediated response to candida and other antigens the patients fail to respond to tuberculin and dinitrochlorobenzene. There is a high incidence in this group of malignant lymphoreticular neoplasms.

GROUP III

i. *Familial chronic mucocutaneous candidosis*: In these patients who develop candidosis in childhood and for whom there is evidence of a recessive autosomal inheritance oral and ungal candidosis is well marked but other sites may be involved.

The most striking associated abnormality in the majority of cases is iron deficiency, usually without anaemia: although the patients apparently absorb iron normally they have difficulty in filling iron stores and the possibility of a genetically determined abnormality of iron metabolism is being investigated. There may also be a deficiency of cellular immune responsiveness, of varying types, to candida.

Similar abnormalities of iron metabolism and immunity may occur in subgroups (ii) and (iii).

ii. In this group of patients the susceptibility to infection other than candida and the exuberant cellular reaction, both of epithelium and connective tissue, are unexplained.

iii. In the late onset group the candidosis is generally limited to the oral cavity and is not seen before the age of 35 years.

In all these patients iron therapy (possibly parenteral), topical antifungal treatment (occasionally systemic) and attempts to induce immune responsiveness by transfer factor or transfusion of lymphocytes have proved useful. In some reduction of antigenic load and iron therapy have restored immunological competence.

None of these forms of chronic mucocutaneous candidosis is associated with an increased incidence of oral squamous-cell carcinoma. The oral features are of chronic thrush—oral epithelial hyperplasia as in chronic hyperplastic candidosis is not seen.

Tuberculosis

This disease is now becoming uncommon due to the improved health of the population and the introduction of specific chemotherapy from 1949 onward. The mouth is only exceptionally involved in the infection in one of four ways:
1. Primary complex.
2. Oral ulceration secondary to open pulmonary tuberculosis.
3. Oral lupus vulgaris.
4. Periapical infection and osteomyelitis.

1. *Aetiology and pathology*

The causative organism is a Gram-positive rod, both acid and alcohol fast, which excites a relatively specific pathological response with epithelioid cells and giant cells with tissue necrosis (caseation). Organisms are present in the lesions where they are demonstrable by the Ziehl–Neelsen technique, they may also be cultured or allowed to proliferate in guinea pigs. Past or present infection is associated with a positive tuberculin test of which the Heaf test is easy to perform and reliable, but the Mantoux test may be employed. Primary infection is associated with a small or completely inconspicuous lesion at the site of entry of the bacillus but marked involvement of the regional lymph nodes. Such a primary complex may occur in the oropharyngeal region, the ileocaecal region or the lung (Ghon focus). Such primary infection may be self-limited or spread widely through the bloodstream. Secondary infection occurs typically in the lung and is a progressive, destructive lesion in a person sensitized to the organism but with some degree of resistance. From such a lesion metastatic infection may occur, particularly in the kidney or in bones.

Clinical features

The typical primary complex in the oropharyngeal region is a completely inconspicuous site of entry with tuberculous cervical lymphadenitis. The organisms frequently gain access through the tonsil but may do so through the mouth and exceptionally an oral ulcer develops at the site of entry. Such cases are common only in children but may occur in adults. The disease presents as an indolent progressive painless ulcer which extends from the gum margin often to the depths of the adjacent vestibule. There is marked regional lymphadenopathy, the glands being firm and matted together and caseation may ensue in them. The Heaf test is positive; blood examination shows no abnormality except raised sedimentation rate. Biopsy of the ulcer reveals the characteristic histological features of tuberculosis and the organism may be demonstrable with Ziehl–Neelsen stain.

Full antituberculous regimen is indicated and the cervical lymph nodes may require aspiration or excision if caseation occurs.

2. Oral ulceration secondary to open pulmonary tuberculosis

Rare, occurring in about 0·2 per cent of such cases and is frequently associated with laryngeal or pharyngeal lesions. Open tuberculosis hence oral lesions is now a disease of the aged or of vagrants. It is particularly important not to exclude the possibility of extensive tuberculosis in such patients because of lack of suggestive symptoms. In the elderly even miliary tuberculosis may be asymptomatic. Usual symptoms, however, include cough, haemoptysis, dyspnoea, weight loss, fever, night sweats and malaise.

The oral ulcer most frequently occurs on the tongue, rarely on the alveolus. It is painful and progressive with a greyish base and sloping edges. Regional lymph nodes are not enlarged. Diagnosis is effected by biopsy and treatment is that of the underlying lesion.

3. Oral lupus vulgaris

This is excessively rare and occurs only in association with extensive lupus on the skin. The oral lesion is an indurated granular or nodular lesion.

4. Periapical tuberculosis and osteomyelitis

In cases of advanced pulmonary tuberculosis the organisms may colonize the periapical granuloma associated with carious teeth and roots and exceptionally this may lead to a 'cold' dento-alveolar abscess. It is said that removal of infected teeth in such patients should be performed soon after the diagnosis is made and with extraction should be carried out curettage of the periapical granuloma.

Tuberculous osteomyelitis is excessively rare and is associated with widespread lesions in the body. It is clinically indistinguishable from chronic suppurative osteomyelitis.

Syphilis

This infection, due to *Treponema pallidum*, is transmitted by sexual intercourse or, rarely, by extragenital mucosal contact, since the organism can neither survive outside the body nor penetrate intact skin. An infected mother may transmit the disease to her fetus, via the placenta, after the first 16 weeks of pregnancy. As a curiosity, the disease may be transmitted in blood transfusion or through a wound in the skin. The incidence of the disease is rising rapidly.

Aetiology and pathology

Treponema pallidum is a small spirochaete about 5–15 μm × 0·25 μm in size with 9–12 tightly wound spirals. It is so fine as to be invisible by light microscopy unless impregnated by silver salts or viewed by reflected light (dark ground illumination) which reveals its active gyrations. The organism cannot be cultured but apparently produces no toxin. The site of entry of the organism into the body is marked by an infiltration of macrophages and lymphocytes but being on mucosae it rapidly ulcerates. This chancre is associated with marked enlargement of the regional lymph nodes. Widespread dissemination of the organism occurs at this stage and the secondary state is characterized by lesions at any site but visible only on the skin and accessible mucosae, although lymphadenopathy is usual. In the final tertiary stage of syphilis the typical pathological lesion is an area of ischaemic necrosis with surrounding fibrosis due to proliferative endarteritis of local blood vessels. The lesions so produced are termed gummata and a similar pathological lesion is the basis of meningo-vascular syphilis and syphilitic aortitis, which is associated with aortic aneurysm, occlusion of the coronary ostia and aortic incompetence. Finally, neurosyphilitic lesions of tabes dorsalis and general paralysis of the insane appear to be due to direct invasion of the nervous system without a vascular basis.

Diagnostic methods in syphilis include:
1. Demonstration of the typical spirochaete.
2. Serological tests.

3. Histopathological examination.

1. Demonstration of the spirochaetes is diagnostic from suspicious genital lesions in the primary and secondary stages. The same does not apply in the mouth, however, due to the indigenous population of treponemes which may be morphologically indistinguishable from *Treponema pallidum*. In a suspicious oral primary lesion the spirochaetes recovered from the enlarged regional lymph nodes, by aspiration, are diagnostic.

2. Serological tests may become positive late in the primary stage but assume great diagnostic importance in the secondary and tertiary stages; they may again become negative in neurosyphilis (but are then positive in CSF). The tests include screening tests—the Wassermann, Khan and Reiter protein complement fixation test and specific tests which must be used to confirm the diagnosis, namely the *Treponema pallidum* immobilization test and the fluorescent treponemal antibody test. Harris (1967) has given a good account of their practical use and interpretation.

3. Histological evidence may provide a guide to the diagnosis in primary oral lesions but is of diagnostic importance only in tertiary syphilis.

Clinical features

These will be considered under the headings congenital and acquired (primary, secondary and tertiary).

A. **Prenatal Syphilis:** The hallmarks of this are:
   a. Interstitial keratitis.
   b. Cochlear degeneration.
   c. Dental abnormalities—Hutchinson's incisors and Moon's molars.
   d. Rhagades.
   e. Depressed nasal bridge.
   f. Childhood gummata.
   g. Juvenile tabes and general paresis.

The dental abnormalities are seen in the incisors and first molars and the typical deformity is a tooth of which the greatest diameter is at the cervix and the shoulders are rounded on to the incisal (or occlusal) surface. The incisal edge is concave or deeply notched while the occlusal surface of the first molar is knobbly with a poor enamel cover. Rhagades are scars radiating from the vermilion borders of the lips. Interstitial keratitis is the commonest expression of congenital syphilis and may recur at intervals for years, ultimately leading to blindness.

B. Acquired Syphilis: Primary oral syphilis is rare and is acquired by orogenital contact or kissing. The oral chancre is painless and is associated with marked painless enlargement of the regional lymph nodes. On the lip of a chancre is a relatively inconspicuous lesion; at first a small papule, it may ulcerate to form a shallow indolent ulcer which is not indurated. Within the mouth the chancre assumes a more florid appearance presenting as a swelling which is bright red with a glossy surface and possibly some ulceration, and closely resembles the pyogenic granuloma or the peripheral reparative granuloma. It is distinguished by the marked non-tender regional lymphadenopathy. Definitive diagnosis is made by examination of fluid from the nodes and in the latter stages, after 10 days, serological tests may become positive.

Secondary syphilis develops 6–8 weeks after innoculation and is characterized by mucous patches associated with fever, generalized lymphadenopathy, skin rash, painless laryngitis and anogenital condylomata (florid soft warty excrescences). All the lesions are highly infectious. The mucous patches which occur on all mucous surfaces are slightly raised, soft whitish lesions which slowly enlarge in a snailtrack fashion. In addition there may be little areas of inflammation which extend to the pharynx. This secondary stage may extend for up to two years. Serological tests are always strongly positive and histology of lesions stained by silver impregnation techniques reveals spirochaetes.

Tertiary syphilitic manifestations follow the original infection by many years and in the mouth these are syphilitic glossitis and gummata.

Syphilitic glossitis is due to obliterative endarteritis which leads to atrophy of the papillae and fissuring due to muscle necrosis and fibrosis. Superimposed upon this are epithelial hyperplasia or dyskeratosis expressed clinically as leucoplakia. The combination of atrophy, leucoplakia and fissuring is not seen in any other condition. Dyskeratosis is present in a high percentage of syphilitic leucoplakias and carcinoma develops in perhaps 20 per cent of cases (although with the overall reduction in the incidence of tertiary syphilis, this specific glossitis is associated with only a small number of lingual cancers).

Gummata commonly occur in the midline of the tongue or palate. Initially, they form indurated swellings but with necrosis there follows ulceration which leads, in the tongue, to a deep painless, indurated, 'punched-out' ulcer with an ischaemic slough in the base and, in the palate, to perforation. In either case serological tests are positive.

There may be associated aortitis (aneurysm, myocardial ischaemia and aortic incompetence), meningovascular syphilis or other gummata, while later tabes dorsalis or general paralysis of the insane predominate.

Treatment

This should be ideally in the hands of a venereologist since proper contact tracing may then be performed. Penicillin is specifically treponemocidal and is the treatment of choice, but heavy metals may also be indicated; penicillin is given as procaine penicillin 600 000 IU intramuscularly daily for 10 days. Careful serological and clinical followup is required.

Whooping Cough (Pertussis)

The only commonly seen oral lesion in this disease is a lingual frenular ulcer which occurs due to the protrusion of the tongue in paroxysms of coughing. Sharp lower incisors are an important factor. Little can be done in the way of specific treatment. Usually the ulcer heals as the paroxysms get less violent.

Scarlet Fever

The significance of this condition has changed radically over the last century and is now a rarely seen condition without its previous fearful mortality. Typically the condition follows a streptococcal infection, in many cases a tonsillitis. In susceptible subjects the effects of scarlet fever are produced by erythrogenic toxin.

Within the mouth the tongue becomes covered with a white coating and the fungiform papillae are inflamed and seen as red dots. This appearance of the tongue is described as a 'white strawberry tongue'. Later the fur on the tongue peels off, but the papillae are still inflamed and the tongue is then described as a 'red strawberry tongue'.

Diphtheria

Again fortunately now a rare disease, but once common. True oral features are not seen but the tonsillar lesions may encroach on the oral epithelium with oedema, inflammation and the dark coloured false membrane formed by a bloody discharge. There will be a foetor ex ore and periadenitis giving the patient a bull neck appearance.

Tetanus

This disease is only mentioned because two of its cardinal features involve the face and jaws. Trismus is an early feature in tetanus and persists for a long time. Stiffness occurs in other parts of the body, especially near the site of the injury, and this will differentiate tetanus from all local causes of trismus. The other feature involving the face is the 'risus sardonicus' due to spasm of the facial muscles: the net effect is to draw the angles of the lips down and screw up the rest of the face. This may occur as part of the paroxysms that are a prominent feature of this disease.

Miscellaneous Infestations

Yaws: This is a chronic progressive inflammatory disease due to *Treponema pertenue* which commonly presents on the face. Mucous membrane is usually unaffected but papillary eruptions occur round the lips, nose and eyes. Hideous destruction of tissue follows where the nose and maxilla can be eroded away. Bone becomes exposed and sequestrates. Teeth can be exfoliated as the disease progresses. Where healing occurs there will be scarring with contracture and further deformity.

Malaria: This can be associated with a very severe form of haemorrhagic gingivitis. Fortunately this is rare, as many cases which have been seen in children have terminated fatally. Chronic gingival disease is extremely common in all patients but can be very marked in patients with malaria, especially if associated with poor oral hygiene. Balendra (1957) claims that this is made even worse with specific antimalarial therapy. All of the oral mucosa may be hyperaemic and painful; this especially applies to the tongue. When anaemia is a marked feature of the malaria, the oral features will correspond.

Toxoplasmosis: Toxoplasmosis is usually considered an uncommon disease in the United Kingdom, but Beattie showed that in Lincolnshire 36 per cent of country-dwellers and 22 per cent of town-dwellers had cytoplasmic modifying antibodies to titres of 1 in 16, as demonstrated by the Sabin–Feldman dye test.

About 5 per cent of lymphadenopathies are attributable to toxoplasmosis and 7 per cent of cases originally diagnosed clinically as glandular fever are in reality toxoplasmosis.

There are two forms of toxoplasmosis: congenital and acquired; we are only concerned with the acquired form here. *Toxoplasma gondii* is a protozoan which exists in a proliferative and cystic form. The cysts are very resistant and survive drying, refrigeration and even gastric juice. A large selection of animals commonly found in most countries harbour the organism.

Aetiology

Human infection is assumed to be from animals, cats appear to be an important vector. Most excreta of animals, including saliva, are rich in the protozoa, but very close contact would be needed as the proliferative form of the organism dies very quickly. The cystic form could be injested in milk and raw meat.

Clinical features

A lymphadenopathy is the most common manifestation of the acquired form of toxoplasmosis. This is seen in the same age group as glandular fever. As the first evidence of the lymphadenopathy often is cervical, there has been the temptation to suggest that the mode of infection was through the tonsils or pharynx.

Initially, the patient feels generally unwell with muscle pain, headache and sore throat. The lymphadenopathy may be painless, but is often associated with inflammation around the lymph nodes which makes them tender. Although the cervical lymph nodes are the first to be discovered, there may be evidence of a generalized lymphadenopathy with chest X-ray confirming hilar enlargement. More severe forms of the disease with evidence of involvement of many different organs occurs in tropical countries and there is a definite mortality to this form of the disease. In the United Kingdom, the condition is often so mild that diagnosis is missed initially and only comes to light when investigation is being made for the persistent lymphadenopathy.

In pregnancy there is a definite danger of the disease being passed on to the fetus. The clinical picture of congenital toxoplasmosis differs greatly from the acquired; there is also a much higher mortality and morbidity rate.

Diagnosis

This is usually confirmed by serology:

1. The Sabin–Feldman dye test which becomes positive within two weeks of infection, but may be delayed in some cases. The basis of this test is that living toxoplasma normally takes up methylene blue dye, but fails to do so in the presence of toxoplasma antibodies, which are found in the patient's serum. Difficulty arises in deciding what level is significant; although patients who are definitely infected may have titres of more than 1 in 1000, levels of 1 in 256 or over are significant.

2. Complement-fixation tests are available, but even here the question of interpretation has difficulties. Levels of 1 in 10 are usually taken as significant.

Other methods of diagnosis have been tried, such as skin tests and biopsy of lymph nodes; neither are entirely satisfactory. Positive information from a biopsy depends on the presence of toxoplasma cysts in the lymph node. Although there is no doubt about the diagnosis when these are found, they are only present in a small percentage of cases.

Treatment

This is far from satisfactory as the drugs available do not always eradicate the toxoplasma and are toxic. Pyrimethamine (Daraprim) is reported to be effective and is given with sulphonamides. It must be remembered that pyrimethamine is a folic acid antagonist and may induce a macrocytic anaemia. To give folic acid with pyrimethamine would neutralize its effect against the toxoplasma. With very mild attacks it is doubtful if treatment is needed.

Bibliography
Actinomycosis

Bramley P. and Orton H. S. (1960) Cervico-facial actinomycosis. *Br. Dent. J.* **109**, 235.
Hertz J. (1957) Actinomycosis. *J. Int. Coll. Surg.* **28**, 539.
Holm P. (1948) Some investigations into the penicillin sensitivity of human pathogenic actinomycetes. *Acta Pathol. Scand.* **25**, 376.
Holmes P. E. B. (1958) Cervico-facial actinomycosis in relation to dental treatment. *Br. Dent. J.* **104**, 314.
Johnson et al. (1957) Actinomycosis of the mandible. *U.S. Armed Forces Med. J.* **8**, 1214.
Mitchell R. G. (1966) Actinomycosis and the dental abscess. *Br. Dent. J.* **120**, 423.
O'Mahoney J. B. (1966) The use of tetracycline in the treatment of actinomycosis. *Br. Dent. J.* **120**, 23.
Rud J. (1967) Cervico-facial actinomycosis. *J. Oral Surg.* **25**, 229.

Fusospirochaetal infections

Blake G. C. (1967) The microbiology of acute ulcerative gingivitis with reference to the culture of oral trichomonads and spirochaetes. *Proc. R. Soc. Med.* **61**, 131.
Emslie R. D. (1963) Cancrum oris. *Dent. Pract.* **13**, 481.
Goldharber P. and Giddon D. B. (1964) The present concepts concerning the aetiology and treatment of acute necrotising ulcerative gingivitis. *Int. Dent. J.* **14**, 468.
Listgarten M. A. (1965) Electron microscopic observations on the bacterial flora of acute necrotising ulcerative gingivitis. *J. Periodontol.* **36**, 328.

Manson J. D. and Rand H. (1961) Recurrent Vincent's disease. *Br. Dent. J.* **110**, 386.
Shinn D. L. S., Squires S. and McFadzean A. (1965) The treatment of Vincent's disease with metronidazole. *Dent. Pract.* **25**, 275.

Candidosis

Budtz–Jorgensen E. (1971) Denture stomatitis IV: an experimental model in monkeys. *Acta Odontol. Scand.* **29**, 513.
Cahn L. (1936) The denture sore mouth. *Ann. Dent.* **3**, 33.
Cawson R. A. (1966) Chronic oral candidiasis and leukoplakia. *Oral Surg.* **22**, 582.
Di George (1965) *Arch. Paediatr.* **67**, 907.
Hermans P. E. and Rittz R. E. (1970) Chronic mucocutaneous candidosis. *Minn. Med.* **53**, 75.
Higgs J. M. and Wells R. S. (1972) Chronic mucocutaneous candidiasis. *Br. J. Dermatol.* **86**, Suppl. 18. 88.
Jepsen A. and Winther J. E. (1965) Mycotic infection in oral leukoplakia. *Acta Odontol. Scand.* **23**, 239.
Lehner T. (1967) Oral candidosis. *Dent. Pract.* **17**, 209.
Neill D. J. and Cawson R. A. (1965) Symposium on Denture Sore Mouth. *Dent. Pract.* **16**, 135.
Winner H. I. and Hurley R. (1964) *Candida Albicans.* London, Churchill.

Tuberculosis

Brand T. A. and Ballard C. F. (1951) Primary tuberculosis of the gum. *Arch. Dis. Child.* **26**, 261.
Cawson R. A. (1960) Tuberculosis of the mouth and throat. *Br. J. Dis. Chest* **54**, 40.
Meng C. M. (1940) Tuberculosis of the mandible. *J. Bone Jt Surg.* **22**, 17.
O'Neill R. (1963) Primary tuberculous ulceration of the gum in an adult. *Br. Dent. J.* **111**, 330.

Syphilis

Bradlaw R. V. (1953) The dental stigmata of prenatal syphilis. *Oral Surg.* **6**, 147.
Harris M. (1967) The serological diagnosis of syphilis. *Br. J. Oral Surg.* **4**, 235.
Meyer I. and Shklar G. (1967) The oral manifestations of acquired syphilis. *Oral Surg.* **23**, 45.
Steiner M. and Alexander W. N. (1966) Primary syphilis of the gingiva. *Oral Surg.* **21**, 530.

Malaria

Balendra (1975) Oral lesions in tropical diseases. Paper read at the International Dental Congress.

Chapter 5

White Lesions of the Oral Mucosa

Introduction

White lesions are due to the appearance of keratinized epithelium at sites in which the epithelium is not normally keratinized, or of excessive keratinization in areas normally keratinized. 'Whiteness' may also be associated with intercellular oedema and accumulation of chronic inflammatory cells. If the term 'leucoplakia' is to be used there must be clear distinction as to its meaning. The indiscriminate use of this term as synonymous for a white patch in the mouth, an area of keratosis, a premalignant lesion or a histological entity, can only lead to confusion. Leucoplakia means a white patch (Greek *leucos*, white; *plakos*, block) and would within these terms of reference legitimately be used for lichen planus or even oral candidosis. The term is best abandoned, as it adds nothing to the diagnosis or description of the lesion and can lead to confusion or even gross mismanagement of the case. A far better nomenclature would be one which gives some indication of the nature of the lesion and its aetiology, e.g. smoker's keratosis, frictional keratosis, etc. There will, of course, be cases under this scheme in which the aetiology is not clear and the lesion has to be called idiopathic keratosis.

Not all mucosa reacts in the same way to harmful stimuli—while some patients produce florid keratosis to minor stimuli, others do not react even to gross insult. Many patients are totally unaware of their lesions until attention is drawn to them. They will be considered under the following headings.

Fordyce Spots

These are ectopic sebaceous glands of the oral mucosa seen in almost every individual but sometimes thought to be abnormal by the novitiate. In fact Fordyce described cases in which masses of glands occurred in the lips (this is seen rather rarely), he knew that occurrence on the buccal

72

mucosa was normal and therefore not noteworthy. Individual glands are yellowish, subepithelial and with a 'diploid' appearance.

Leucoedema

This is an ill-defined condition and the term is merely a description of the appearance of the oral mucosa, which is whitish-grey in colour and looks over-hydrated. The mucosa usually has a slightly wrinkled surface and if it is stretched the lesion tends to disappear or to become reticulated. Histologically there is some increased keratin but very little difference from the white sponge naevus. Usually the condition is seen as a casual observation and is of no significance. A higher incidence of leucoedema is seen among those of African or Asiatic descent, indeed among American Negroes there appears to be an increasing incidence among children until in adults the majority (50–90 per cent) are affected. Pindborg describes leucoedema occurring bilaterally in a high percentage of betel nut chewers.

Diagnosis is important so that the patient can be spared repeated biopsy and surgery.

'White Sponge Naevus'

This is a diffuse developmental keratotic lesion of the mucosal surfaces which is completely benign and often hereditary.

Synonyms: The large number of names used in this field reflects the confusion that has reigned in connection with this condition. Cannon introduced the term 'white sponge naevus' in 1935, but even the white appearance is not a constant feature. Other terms used are: congenital leucokeratosis mucosa oris, hereditary leucokeratosis (white mouth), pachyderma oralis, white folded gingivostomatosis, familial white folded hypertrophy of mucous membrane, oral epthelial naevi.

Pachyonychia congenita and hereditary benign intra-epithelial dyskeratosis are considered separately by some authors, but they have to admit that histologically and clinically there is little to distinguish these two conditions from the white sponge naevus. The problem is to find a name which describes the clinical and histological appearances accurately. None is really satisfactory. Hereditary factors have been shown in some cases, even to the point of suggesting that in these cases the condition is inherited as an autosomal dominant. Other cases seem to appear spontaneously as a congenital condition without a family history. Even the congenital aspect of this condition is disputed in many cases where it was either missed at earlier examinations or became more prominent later in life. As would be expected, there is no age or sex incidence. In all cases the condition is symptomless.

Clinical features

Although the oral mucosa is usually involved, lesions may occur in the nose, pharynx, oesophagus, rectum and anus. Genital lesions have been described on the labia of the vulva, the vagina and the glans penis. In the mouth the buccal mucosa is most commonly affected, but the tongue, floor of the mouth, palate, labial mucosa and even the gingiva may be involved. Usually the lesions are bilateral. The mucosa may appear diffusely keratotic with an opalescent appearance. It may be thrown into folds which have been poetically described as looking like the sand after the ebbing of the tide. Alternatively, the mucosa may appear thickened, spongy or even shaggy. The fact that the surface keratin can often be removed with dry gauze has frequently led to the condition being wrongfully diagnosed as oral candidosis and even to its being treated with antifungal agents. It is only the spongy case which lives up to the name of white sponge naevus.

Differential diagnosis

The importance of making a correct diagnosis is to prevent the patient being treated for some other condition. Once the diagnosis has been established, it is important to explain the condition to the patient in the best possible terms, for his own protection.

The condition can be confused with keratosis, but usually the history makes the distinction clear, although cheek biting, frictional keratosis and snuff or tobacco chewers' keratosis all have a similar appearance. Leucoedema also has a very similar appearance until the mucosa is stretched. Darier–White's disease, although hereditary, usually gives rise to cutaneous lesions as well as mucosal lesions. It should only rarely be necessary to subject the patient to syphilitic serological and biopsy examinations, but this should be done once in any case where there is doubt.

Course and prognosis

The white spongy naevus is a completely benign lesion which remains static and symptomless throughout life. It is best to leave the condition well alone after informing the patient of its nature and its hereditary implications.

Darier–White's Disease: This very rare condition was described simultaneously by both Darier and White in 1889. Darier called the condition 'psorospermose folliculaire vegetante' and White described the same condition as 'keratosis (ichthyosis) follicularis'.

Keratosis is first seen in childhood, with small keratotic patches on the head, neck, back, chest, abdomen and especially in the groin and axillae. The hands and feet are covered with numerous small lesions on their palmar and plantar surfaces. Verrucous keratotic patches are to be seen in the mouth and other mucosal surfaces. Malignant changes are not described, but infection may occur round the skin lesions and this can cause follicular obstruction. White lesions may occur in the mouth in other rare inherited disorders of epithelium including dyskeratosis congenita and pachonychia congenita.

Frictional Keratosis (including lip and cheek biting)

Most of the younger patients with frictional keratosis are women who habitually bite their cheeks or lips. This type of lesion is not confined to the female sex, but is seen quite often in young teenage girls, some of whom may continue to bite their cheek while giving their history, claiming that they are unable to stop themselves. The area of mucosa affected appears rough and greyish-white and the distribution is characteristic, extending inside the lower lip and then back along the occlusal line on both sides. Usually the patient gives up the habit spontaneously, but often not before there has been some dark pigmentation due to chronic haemorrhagic lesions in the submucosa.

Patients with minor malocclusions often nip the buccal mucosa of the cheek along the occlusal line. This is a remarkably constant feature of temporomandibular joint dysfunction. A line may be seen in one or both cheeks where the teeth occlude, often with indentations for individual teeth. The tongue is frequently involved in this type of patient, with a small white area on the lateral margin, sometimes in relation to an instanding tooth.

Patients with missing teeth often have an area of keratosis on the gum that is acting instead of a tooth and is thus being stimulated beyond its physiological limits. A denture can cause trauma to the mucosa, especially if it has badly placed clasps which impinge on adjacent mucosa.

Treatment

The treatment of this condition is simply to remove the aetiological factor. If it is a sharp tooth, this should be made smooth and functional dentures constructed where needed. Patients with cheek-biting habits will present a problem and usually resist treatment or suggestion that they should abandon their habit. To fight with them over this only makes the condition worse. Usually the senseless habit is abandoned and only the more persistent cases will present as a problem. There is a parallel between this condition and nail-biting.

Tobacco-related Keratosis

This is one of the most common causes of keratosis in the mouth. Patients often have poor oral hygiene and are in the fifth or sixth decade of life. Males are much more frequently affected than females and there seems to be a correlation between the amount smoked and the number and severity of the lesions.

In pipe smokers the lesions are commonly on the palate. There may be a focal area of keratosis where the smoke of the pipe plays on the mucosa. Some patients keep their pipe in one set position, while others move it from side to side. Facets may be worn in the teeth which coincide with the position of the pipe. Usually the teeth are heavily coated with a brown to black tar deposit on the lingual and palatal surfaces. If the patient wears an upper denture with palatal covering the mucosa will be protected although the denture will be heavily stained.

Focal lesions appear as discrete white plaques, but may be tessellated, with a surrounding margin of erythematous mucosa. The rest of the mucosa of the palate may have a whitish appearance. Mucosal ducts can appear as red dots and on the posterior part of the palate as red dots surrounded by a white keratotic ring. This may give a rough appearance which occasionally is appreciated by the patient. This appearance is called stomatitis nicotina.

In cigarette smokers the changes in the mouth are usually more diffuse. The buccal mucosa of the cheeks has a milky white appearance which is more pronounced at the commissures, fading in the molar region. Changes may be seen on the mucosal surface of the lips and tongue and more rarely on the floor of the mouth. Patients who leave a cigarette hanging on their lip often have a groove worn which may be keratinized. Heavy cigarette smokers have nicotine-stained fingers unless they use a holder and even a grey moustache or beard will have a brownish-yellow discoloration.

Cigar smokers quickly develop stomatitis nicotina and nicotine-stained teeth, but little keratosis. This is because cigar smokers generally smoke less than cigarette or pipe smokers.

Pindborg reviewed the smoking habits he found in parts of India, Papua and New Guinea and related them to white lesions in the mouth. He commented on the high incidence of these lesions among bidi smokers. Bidi is a cheap form of cigarette made by rolling a piece of dried, tender leaf with a locally grown tobacco of varying type secured between the folds of the leaf with a thread. Over 15 per cent of all bidi smokers had areas of keratosis.

Clinical course

Although malignant changes are rare in case of frictional keratosis, this is not always the case with smokers' keratosis. Many patients have slowly developed lesions over the years with little symptomatology. Others may have noticed a dry sensation in the mouth only relieved by a further cigarette. Eventually there will be cacogeusia, but on some occasions the taste is impaired. Most smokers have a characteristic odour of the breath which can be quite objectionable to non-smokers.

Treatment

Because of the danger of malignant changes, patients should be encouraged to stop smoking or at least to cut down the amount they smoke. This counsel of perfection is often difficult to implement, as most people who smoke enjoy the habit. It can even be claimed that there are addictive qualities about smoking, although it is doubtful if enough nicotine is absorbed. Nicotine in small doses is a CNS stimulant in that it acts as the transmitting agent at autonomic ganglia. Large doses of nicotine would cause autonomic blockade by depolarization, but such doses are never reached even in the heaviest of smokers. Many smokers claim that they are capable of higher levels of thought while smoking. This claim must be regarded with suspicion.

Unfortunately smoking is a socially acceptable habit, giving idle hands an occupation and providing a slight distraction which can be very convenient in speech. The mere offering of cigarettes or cigars has become a token of hospitality or friendship.

From the health aspect there can be little defence of smoking. In the United Kingdom 25 000 people die each year from carcinoma of the bronchus, to say nothing of the bronchitis which is perpetuated. Vascular disease is probably accelerated by smoking with a higher incidence of myocardial infarction. Peptic ulceration is potentiated by smoking and there are reports that women who smoke during pregnancy give birth to smaller babies.

Oral lesions may be only a small factor, but even so, they often provide the patient with a useful chance to give up smoking. Time is well spent in explaining the situation to the patient, for when presented with the facts the sensible patient will want to cooperate and usually asks advice on abandoning his habit.

Alteration in smoking habits may help some patients. A change to the occasional cigar is very useful, especially in female patients, as cigar smoking is not universally acceptable for ladies. Lobeline as a replacement for nicotine has been tried, either as lobeline sulphate 2 mg (in Lobidan) or lobeline hydrochloride 1 mg (in Lobron Anti-smoking Pastilles). Unfortunately neither is completely successful on its own, but may be useful as an adjunct in a willing patient. Initially patients will have to learn to avoid the circumstances which excite the desire to smoke, such as travelling in the smoking compartment of a train with other active smokers, or in the company of friends who will offer them cigarettes and ridicule their efforts to stop smoking. Basically it is the underlying personality which will decide the success or failure of the treatment, and as with any reformed addict, the relapse rate will be high. Some patients become discouraged because their cessation of smoking causes an increase in appetite and consequent weight gain.

In certain patients where reference has been made to the potential dangers of malignant disease, smoking may be substituted by a cancer phobia. A number of patients are being seen who arrive at hospital with a cancer phobia due to a practitioner having observed a white patch in the mouth and having informed the patient that he needs specialist opinion, as the lesion may be malignant. Although fear is the only real deterrent to smoking, the eventual condition may be worse than the first.

Tobacco Chewers' Keratosis: Keratosis can occur in the buccal mucosa, but the incidence is not as high as in patients who have primitive smoking habits. The area of keratosis is usually diffuse.

Oral Snuff Keratosis: Snuff is not always used in the nose; cases are occasionally seen where snuff, which may have various constituents, e.g. powdered tobacco 91 per cent, menthol 4·5 per cent and eucalyptus oil 4·5 per cent, is placed in the lower labial sulcus. This causes a diffuse keratosis and discoloration of the teeth.

Because of the risk of malignancy, none of the above habits should be encouraged—a counsel of perfection in remote parts of the world.

Betel Nut Chewers' Keratosis

Pindborg and his associates have undertaken epidemiological surveys among betel nut chewers. They describe how, in Papua and New Guinea the inhabitants chew the betel nut when it is ripe, but before it is cured. After a few minutes chewing a moist stick is dipped in pulverized slaked lime and this is introduced into the mouth and wiped on the buccal mucosa and licked clean. In India the betel nut is chewed cured or raw with slaked lime and catachu added, the mixture being known as a *pan*. Tobacco may be chewed with *pan*.

As a result of these habits, a diffuse keratosis may occur in the buccal mucosa. Where the stick is wiped on the mucosa, a streak of keratosis is seen maximal at the commissure of the mouth. Cases of keratosis may be seen as early as the third decade of life in both men and women who indulge in this habit.

Lichen Planus

Lichen planus is a cutaneous and mucosal disease which is typified by small papular eruptions, but there are many variants, including bullous, atrophic and erosive forms.

Aetiology

No definite aetiological factor can be cited, but the old concept of a viral infection is giving place to supposed psychosomatic factors. This is supported by the fact that lichen planus is more commonly seen in patients with mild anxiety features and occurs associated with increased stress. In spite of this, there are reports of lichenified eruptions occurring following the administration of gold, arsenical compounds, bismuth, mepacrine, chloroquine, hydroxychloroquine, amiphenazole and chlorpropamide.

Incidence

Lichen planus accounts for about 1 per cent of the dermatological conditions seen in the skin clinic. In such cases oral lesions occur in 50–70 per cent of patients, yet only 10 per cent of the cases with oral lesions have associated skin lesions. A wide age group (20–60) is affected with a slightly higher incidence in females.

Clinical features

Cutaneous lesions: The most common lesion is a papular eruption which may be discrete or widespread in the form of a rash. Lesions are classically described as being seen maximally on the flexor surfaces of limbs or where clothes rub. Very often the condition seems to rebel against classical form and can be seen anywhere on the body. There may be a linear pattern which has been said to follow the line of a nerve or a scratch. Alternatively, papules may be arranged to give an annular appearance. The papules may itch intensely, which causes the patient to scratch and so distort the original presentation. Some papules fade quickly, while others persist for months and may leave a small area of pigmentation, probably due to the irritation.

If a little oil is applied to the papules and wiped off again with a piece of dry gauze, the pattern of the lesion can be seen more clearly. With the aid of a hand lens white striae can be seen which were first described by Wickham in 1895 and bear his name. Again with the aid of a lens, the edge of the lesion often appears to be raised. These two points are sometimes diagnostically useful.

Most papules have a silvery to purple appearance but this may be exchanged for an erythematous type of eruption which makes diagnosis more difficult. Bullae are rarely seen, even when they occur they have usually ruptured before the patient presents, leaving non-specific crusted lesions. Atrophic lesions may appear like a healing abrasion but may have Wickham's striae on the surface. Vesicular forms were more commonly seen when arsenic was in use for the treatment of syphilis. In most of these rarer variants a more classical lesion is seen if a careful search is made.

Nails, especially fingernails, are involved in 10 per cent of cases. Usually the damage is mild, giving vertical ridges like depressions, which gradually grow out. Less commonly the nail is more severely damaged, with partial or complete destruction of the nail bed.

Oral manifestations: In the main, patients with oral lichen planus have a high standard of oral hygiene with well-conserved teeth. As on the skin, the most common oral lesion is papular, but atrophic, erosive and occasionally bullous forms are to be seen. Most patients complain of a sore mouth or even a metallic taste with a dry sensation. Some patients are quite unaware of the lesion in the mouth. Commonly the lesions are seen on the buccal mucosa, especially in the third molar region; another common site is the lateral margin of the tongue. More rarely the lesions may be seen on the gingiva and even the mucosal surface of the lips, involvement of the mucosal surface of the lips seems to be characteristic of drug-induced lichen planus. Often the lesions are bilateral and at a number of sites.

Careful examination, perhaps aided by a hand lens, will show that each papule is about 2 mm in diameter (the size of a pinhead) and may be set on an erythematous base. Cooke described in detail the various patterns that can be made by the small papules: a reticular pattern is most characteristic of the condition, this may be incomplete, giving a linear or even an annular appearance. Discrete papules may be multiple and can give the appearance of colonies of *Candida albicans* or papules may become confluent, giving a dense white patch.

When the dorsum of the tongue is involved the lesions tend to involve a broad band down the midline. This is well keratinized with a tessellated surface and atrophy of the papillae.

Atrophic lesions are common with a thin, red and shiny mucosa. This easily breaks down to produce an erosion which takes a very long time to heal; in some cases this may be years. Quite often papules, atrophic areas and erosions all occur together, round the edge of the lesion there may be white papules in various forms, giving place to an atrophic area which has a central erosive area. When the atrophic lesion does finally heal, there is often residual pigmentation. Rarely the lesions are purely ulcerative and very widespread oral ulceration may occur (lesions comparable in extent only occurring in erythema multiforme exudativum); even then it is usually possible to find some papules which allow diagnosis to be made.

Sites of other lesions: Lichen planus, especially in its papular form, is often seen on the glans penis and the vulva. More rarely, it has been described in the nose, rectum and anus. Occasionally it is also seen in the pharynx, larynx, oesophagus and even further down the alimentary tract on gastric mucosa and colon. In the urinary tract it may occasionally be seen in the urethra and the bladder. Cases have been described in which it was present in the ear and on the tympanic membrane.

The clinical features vary with the region involved. Rectal and anal lesions are a possible cause of pruritus ani.

Differential diagnosis of oral lesions

Usually this is a problem of deciding between oral keratosis of the various types and lichen planus, thus this difficulty occurs mostly in the confluent type of lichen planus. Although the history and site or sites of the lesion may help, a biopsy may be the only way of making a final decision. Leucoedema may be mistaken for the coarse reticular lichen planus, especially if the mucosa is lightly stretched while being examined. A reticular pattern may be seen in patients with oral candidosis, but this usually wipes off and if any doubt still exists it should be cultured. Chronic discoid lupus erythematosus may give a static ulcer with some keratosis round the margin. This is often mistaken for lichen planus, unless other features of the disease are present. A biopsy interpreted by a histologist very experienced in oral pathology is often the first clue to this condition. Pemphigus and pemphigoid do not really present a great problem, as the surrounding mucosa is very friable. Severe cases of lichen planus which have eroded can have a friable mucosa. Exfoliative cytology for acantholytic cells (Tzanck cells) or biopsy will be the final court of appeal. Ectopic sebaceous glands (Fordyce's spots) can mimic the papules of lichen planus to the untrained eye.

The Question of Malignant Changes in Lichen Planus

'Malignant changes are extremely rare in lichen planus' was the leading sentence in the first edition. There is, however, increasing evidence that it is commoner than once suspected. The French literature has always emphasized the importance of oral lichen planus as a precancerous lesion.

The surveys of Kovesi and Banoczy have noted 1 case of carcinoma in a series of 274 followed-up patients while carcinoma only seems to supervene in long-standing erosive cases. Personal experience points to a higher figure with the risk of carcinoma at least as great as that in 'idiopathic keratosis'; *see* p. 133.

Treatment

Mild asymptomatic cases without erosion need no treatment, but should be kept under periodic observation for deterioration. These are the very patients who can so easily develop a cancer phobia, as their personality provides the right seed bed. Even a biopsy can be enough to start the patient worrying unnecessarily, to say nothing of incautious discussion. If there are mild oral sensations, all that may be needed is a phenolic and alkaline mouthwash (collut. phenol alk. BPC), 15 ml in a half tumbler of warm water, to be used before and after meals.

Topical steroids are very useful in lichen planus, especially the troublesome erosive form varying the preparation according to the severity of the condition or its persistence. By starting with the weakest preparation and progressing to a stronger, more potent steroids are retained in reserve for the most severe or persistent case.

A useful scheme is to start with hydrocortisone hemisuccinate pellets (Corlan) 2·5 mg qds allowed to dissolve on the lesion. Progression can then be made to 0·1 per cent triamcinolone in an emollient dental base (Adcortyl A in Orabase) qds. If this fails, or the initial lesions are particularly severe, the patient can be started on betamethasone (Beta-Corlan) 0·1 mg qds allowed to dissolve on the lesion. In resistant cases intra-lesional injection of prednisolone phosphate (10 mg) may be useful.

Idiopathic Keratosis

Cases of oral keratosis present where no aetiological factor can be found. When it occurs in older patients it is tempting to call this senile keratosis, but this is not really citing an aetiological factor and these cases would be best included as idiopathic. There must be an aetiological factor(s) not yet apparent. It is known that vitamin A deficiency will result in mucosal keratosis, but there is no evidence of occult vitamin A deficiency in these patients.

The area involved may be single and discrete or there may be a number of areas scattered around the mouth. Some authors have suggested that there is a higher incidence of oral keratosis in patients with an iron deficiency anaemia than in a control sample.

Sublingual 'Butterfly' Keratosis of the Floor of the Mouth

This was originally classified, by Cooke, as a naevus and was assumed to be as innocent as the white sponge naevus. Although it has a similar clinical and histological appearance as the naevus its appearance in late middle age usually in women, its characteristic distribution and propensity for malignant change mark it as an entity worthy of separate consideration.

Clinical features

The lesion has a characteristic butterfly shape in the floor of the mouth, the lesion tends to slowly and progressively expand. The edges are well marked and the surface wrinkled and dead white. It is rarely seen before the age of 40 and is much more common in women, particularly smokers, and tobacco may be significant in the aetiology. The lesion should be observed closely as carcinoma supervenes in a high proportion of cases.

Psoriasis

Psoriatic lesions on the palate, buccal mucosa, lip and tongue have been described. It is only fair to state that there are some authorities who doubt the existence of true psoriasis in the mouth, yet there are a few cases where the diagnosis is backed with histological evidence.

The lesion usually takes the form of a small papule with the appearance of a white plaque. In the absence of histology and typical dermatological lesions, a diagnosis of oral keratosis or lichen planus could quite easily be made. Linear lesions have been described and lesions with more the appearance of snail track syphilitic ulcer.

When the lesion occurs on the vermilion part of the lips, it has a much more characteristic appearance, with definite scaling. If the scales are removed with the fingernail, there will be the typical small bleeding points where subpapillary capillaries have been exposed.

In doubtful cases it may be necessary to biopsy or to wait expectantly. The oral lesions will disappear when the cutaneous lesions go into remission.

Acanthosis Nigricans

There are two principal subgroups to this disorder—an inherited variety and an acquired form which is commonly indicative of internal (gut) malignancy. Some observers subdivide into further groups. In this context it is only necessary to note that in the acquired form oral lesions may rarely appear and have the same significance as the commoner skin lesions. The lesions are somewhat papilliferous like an extensive sessile papilloma, usually on the lip and tongue, with a white surface. The cutaneous lesions are common in the axillae, groins and neck and consist of pigmented papilliferous or tessellated plaques.

Differential diagnosis

In the mouth which shows evidence of heavy smoking, it is not difficult to diagnose smokers' keratosis, but it is in these very circumstances that syphilis could slip by unnoticed.

As the differentiation of the various types of keratosis is made from the aetiology, it is from the history that the differentiation is made, with the exception of syphilitic keratosis, when positive syphilitic serology is the deciding factor. It would be a wise precaution to undertake serology in all cases of oral keratosis. Lichen planus can often be differentiated clinically by the pattern of the lesions, the multi-positional distribution, and the occurrence in a patient with good oral hygiene. Skin lesions may clinch the diagnosis, but can cause even more confusion if they represent some of the subtle variants of lichen planus.

Oral candidosis can be mistaken for keratosis, especially the chronic form often called 'Candida leucoplakia' which, unlike most of the white lesions of oral candidosis, does not wipe off with a piece of gauze. Direct microscopy and culture may reveal *Candida albicans* in the mycelial form, which suggests that the organism is present as a pathogen. *Candida albicans* can be present as a secondary infection of a keratotic area.

The final court of appeal in all white lesions is a biopsy. This may be necessary to distinguish between lichen planus and the various types of keratosis. It is unkind and unnecessary to submit all patients to a biopsy, but it does have the advantage of excluding change in suspect lesions.

To summarize, all patients with white lesions in the mouth should have haemoglobin and serology for syphilis. Some cases will need scrapings for *Candida albicans* and others will need a biopsy.

Many keratotic lesions in the mouth remain benign especially if the aetiological factor is removed. Others will progress to a carcinoma *in situ* only after a long interval and with continued stimulation. Even so, it is true that occasional white lesions are seen which progress very quickly to a squamous-cell carcinoma. Thus all patients must be kept under regular observation, Surgery or radiotherapy should always be undertaken when the lesion has passed to the carcinoma *in situ* stage or further, which can only be proved for certain by biopsy and even then there may be a difference in histological interpretation.

The clinical features which suggest malignant changes are ulceration, erythroplasia, induration and lymphadenopathy. Any keratotic lesion that ulcerates must be considered suspicious. Erosion is common in lichen planus but significant in keratosis. If the lesion loses its white appearance and becomes red and hypertrophic with a nodular appearance it should be biopsied immediately. Induration indicates that there is some extension of the superficial pathology into the deeper tissues, giving the base of the lesion a firm and even attached appearance. This is often the result of malignant changes. Regional lymphadenopathy can be due to other causes, but unless they are very obvious, malignant change in the concurrent oral keratosis must be suspected.

The risks of carcinoma supervening in cases of oral keratosis are considered in Chapter 11.

Bibliography

Leucoedema and white sponge naevus

Cannon A. N. (1935) White sponge naevus of the mucosa. *Arch. Dermatol.* **31**, 365.

Cohen L. and Young A. H. (1968) The white sponge naevus. *Br. J. Oral Surg.* **5**, 206.

Cooke B. E. D. and Morgan J. (1959) Oral epithelial naevi. *Br. J. Dermatol.* **71**, 134.

Darling A. I. and Fletcher J. P. (1958) Familial white folded gingivostomatitis. *Oral Surg.* **11**, 296.

Haye K. R. and Whitehead F. I. H. (1968) Hereditary leukokeratosis of the mucous membrane. *Br. J. Dermatol.* **80**, 529.

Martin J. L. and Crump E. P. (1972) Leukoedema of the buccal mucosa in Negro children and youth. *Oral Surg.* **34**, 49.

Payne T. F. (1975) Why are white lesions white? *Oral Surg.* **40**, 652.

Pindborg J. J. et al. (1968) Epidemiology and histology of oral leukoplakia and leukoedema among Papuans and New Guineans. *Cancer* **22**, 379.

Lichen planus

Andreasen J. O. (1968) Oral lichen planus. *Oral Surg.* **25**, 31.

Cawson R. A. (1968) Treatment of oral lichen planus with betamethasone. *Br. Med. J.* **1**, 86.

Cooke B. E. D. (1954) Oral manifestations of lichen planus: 50 cases. *Br. Dent. J.* **96**, 1.

Darling A. I. and Crabb H. S. M. (1954) Lichen planus. *Oral Surg.* **7**, 1276.

Dechaume, M., Payen J. and Piriou M. (1957) 'Le lichen plan isolé de la muquèse buccale. Considérations anatomo-cliniques d'après 50 observations dont 30 avec examen histologique. *Presse Méd.* **65**, 2133.

Dinsdale R. C. W. and Walker A. E. (1966) Amiphenazole sensitivity with oral ulceration. *Br. Dent. J.* **121**, 460.

Dinsdale R. C. W. et al. (1968) Lichenoid eruption due to chlorpropamide. *Br. Med. J.* **1**, 100.

Kovesi G. and Banoczy J. (1973) Follow-up studies in oral lichen planus. *Oral Surg.* **2**, 13.

Saurat J. H. et al. (1975) The lichen planus like eruption after bone-marrow transplantation. *Br. J. Dermatol.* **92**, 675.

Silverman S. and Griffith M. (1974) Studies on oral lichen planus. II. Follow-up on 200 patients, clinical characteristics and associated malignancy. *Oral Surg.* **37**, 705.

Warin R. P. et al. (1958) Lichen planus of the mouth. *Br. Med J.* **1**, 983.

Other white lesions

Cooke B. E. D. (1956) Leukoplakia buccalis and oral epithelial naevi—a clinical and histological study. *Br. J. Dermatol.* **68,** 151.

Kramer I. R. H., Labban N. and Lee K. W. (1978) The clinical features and risk of malignant transformation in sublingual keratosis, *Br. Dent. J.* **144,** 171.

Pindborg J. J. et al. (1968) Epidemiology and histology of oral leukoplakia and leukoedema among Papuans and New Guineans. *Cancer* **22,** 379.

Pindborg J. J. et al. (1967) Studies in oral leukoplakias. *Bull. WHO* **37,** 109.

Pisanty S. and Ship I. I. (1970) Oral psoriasis. *Oral Surg.* **30,** 351.

Witkop C. J. and Gorlin R. J. (1961) Four hereditary mucosal syndromes. *Arch. Dermatol.* **84,** 762.

Chapter 6

Miscellaneous Mucosal Lesions

Uraemia

In uraemia, of any cause, there may develop a painful chemical stomatitis which seriously interferes with the nutrition of the patient and hence management of the underlying disease.

Pathogenesis

The lesion is probably due to the metabolism of salivary urea by oral bacterial urease with production of ammonia. It is particularly associated with poor oral hygiene and periodontal disease and especially supragingival calculus, and does not occur in the edentulous. Paradoxically, the stomatitis only occurs in a small percentage of patients and when it does occur it is not related directly to the severity of the condition as judged by the blood urea, but tends to occur in advanced cases. It is particularly troublesome during the diuretic phase of acute renal failure when the need for oral potassium supplements may be present, as these are particularly painful on the damaged mucosa.

Clinical features

The patient complains of a sore mouth and examination reveals diffuse inflammation with loss of superficial epithelium leading to an atrophic appearance of the epithelium. The characteristic lesion is, however, a wrinkled white plaque of coagulated surface epithelium which usually occurs in the floor of the mouth, labial sulcus or tongue. Non-specific ulceration may occur.

Treatment

In the first place, careful oral hygiene is important with removal of the tartar and careful cleansing of the teeth. The mouth is rinsed with hydrogen peroxide (10 volume) diluted with an equal volume of water. This is quite acid. Subsequently, the lesions are painted with Compound Crystal Violet Paint BPC. Treatment is carried out four times daily.

Lupus Erythematosus

This condition exists in two forms, the localized form known as chronic discoid lupus erythematosus and systemic lupus erythematosus where there are features involving almost every organ of the body. On occasions it may be very difficult to decide into which of the two groups the cases should be included.

In systemic lupus erythematosus (SLE) oral lesions can occur in up to a quarter of patients. This condition is usually confined to females in the child-bearing age group. Rashes and lymphadenopathy are the most common presenting signs, but frequently there is evidence of renal, hepatic, pulmonary or nervous system involvement. The rash is classically maculopapular and typically occurs on the face, especially the cheeks. There is some degree of photosensitivity, which may cause the cutaneous lesions to become bullous.

Purpuric areas appear on the gingiva, palate and even in other areas. These tend to group together and break down to form a painful ulcer. Lesions may extend into the pharynx, making eating and swallowing very painful. Secondary infection, as always, makes the condition much worse.

In chronic discoid lupus erythematosus, oral lesions do not occur in such a high proportion of cases. The solitary oral lesion is rarely seen and presents a difficult diagnostic problem. Lips, tongue and buccal mucosa can all be involved. There is considerable variation in the type of lesion ranging from an atrophic area of mucosa with a tendency to ulcerate, surrounded by a margin of hyperkeratosis, to areas of extensive ulceration, with crusting, and finally healing with scar formation.

Visually the differential diagnosis of chronic lupus erythematosus is from erosive lichen planus, keratosis with ulceration and even in some cases of acute onset from erythema multiforme. A biopsy will do much to clarify the position, but there will be many cases where the histology is not diagnostic. Simultaneous appearance of cutaneous lesions does much to help in making a positive diagnosis.

Many cases of chronic discoid lupus erythematosus will show laboratory features of systematization and the following investigations should be undertaken.

Haemoglobin: there may be anaemia.

White cell count: there may be leukopenia.
Platelets: there may be thrombocytopenia.
ESR may be raised.
Plasma proteins: the serum globulin may be raised.
LE cells may be found.
Antinuclear factor may be positive.
Rheumatoid factor may be positive.
Serology for syphilis may be positive.
There may be a positive direct Coombs' test.

Only a very small percentage of cases of discoid lupus erythematosus proceed to systemic lupus erythematosus, in spite of the high percentage of cases with laboratory features of more diffuse disease.

Treatment of systemic lupus erythematosus obviously comes outside the scope of this book. The oral lesions of discoid lupus erythematosus are best treated with topical steroids. Triamcinolone 0·1 per cent in an emollient dental base (Adcortyl in Orabase) is very useful. Alternatively 0·1 mg pellets of betamethasone (Beta Corlan) may be sucked four times a day. Lesions may be very resistant to treatment requiring considerable perseverence both on the part of the patient and the clinician. For this reason, care should be exercised over prolonged use of betamethasone as considerable amounts of steroid are absorbed. In extremely recalcitrant cases it may be necessary to resort to systemic chloroquine derivatives or gold injections. Both these treatments carry their dangers and are best avoided where other means will suffice.

Hypersensitivity Reactions

Only the immediate or anaphylactic (Type I) and delayed type (Type IV) hypersensitivity responses occur in the mouth. Angio-oedema represents the Type I reaction and fixed drug eruptions together with contact hypersensitivity represent the Type IV.

Angio-oedema: There is still a great deal of mystery surrounding this condition. Even the name is misleading, suggesting a defective neuromuscular response which is one of the few definite mechanisms that has been shown to be normal. As there are two types of this condition, there are in all probability at least two mechanisms. The hereditary type is a serious inherited (dominant) condition in which there is absence of a specific enzyme inhibitor of complement C_1 esterase, thus activation of the complement system as a result of minor stimuli which would normally not trigger a response may occur and trauma, very commonly the result of dental treatment, may provide such a stimulus. This results in localized swelling which can be hazardous to life with many patients dying of laryngeal obstruction.

Recurrent abdominal pain is an important clinical feature. Amelioration of the swelling may be produced by antifibrinolytic agents (tranexamic acid being the drug of choice) given before dental or surgical treatment. In the event of laryngeal oedema subcutaneous adrenaline or cricothyrotomy (or tracheostomy) may be indicated.

The *non-hereditary* type of angio-oedema has an allergic basis. Often the condition occurs in patients who have a history of urticarial reactions or other allergies. An initial antigen produces sensitizing antibodies called reagins which will react with the mast cells of skin of mucosa. On subsequent challenge by an antigen there is immediate release of 5-hydroxytryptamine, kinins and histamine from the mast cells. The result is oedema of subcutaneous or submucosal tissue which may affect any part of the body especially the eyelids, lips, tongue and even the tissue planes of the floor of the mouth, which may lead to laryngeal oedema. Even though this is called the non-hereditary type of angio-oedema, it would appear that the ability to form reagin is an inherited factor, but does not always result in angioneurotic oedema; it may give rise to hay fever, asthma, urticaria and anaphylactic shock.

Clinically there is a wide range of severity from mild non-consequential localized swelling to widespread oedema. As the condition often occurs as indicated above in the head and neck, the picture is of a patient with a red bloated face, lips and eyelids. Swallowing may be embarrassed and so may respiration. At this stage patients become frightened and are usually admitted sitting up fighting for breath. Cyanosis is a very ominous clinical feature signifying that a dramatic asphyxial termination is about to occur.

This condition must be treated as a medical emergency in hospital. Large doses of intravenous hydrocortisone should be given, doses of 200 mg are minimal and no harm will come from high doses such as 500 mg. Subcutaneous 1:1000 adrenaline has a useful place provided there is no tachycardia exceeding 120 per minute. One ml of 1:1000 adrenaline may be drawn up in a syringe, the needle inserted subcutaneously and half given slowly immediately and the rest after a few minutes. Large doses of antihistamines are given intramuscularly such as 50 mg of promethazine hydrochloride. Oxygen will help to decrease the hypoxia and cyanosis, but if the airway is completely blocked an emergency tracheostomy is a life-saving procedure.

Even when the patient's condition is satisfactory initially or becomes satisfactory after medical treatment, very careful observations need to be maintained on the patient. Nurses must be instructed on physical signs indicative of deterioration. Steroids and antihistamines may need to be continued for a few days, and in recurrent cases antihistamines may need to continue for months. In these cases, bearing in mind the possible serious consequences, the precipitating factor should be found and an effort made to desensitize the patient.

Fixed Drug Eruption: It is rare for a fixed drug eruption to occur in the mouth. The most common drug to cause this is phenolphthalein which is often the basic ingredient of proprietary purgatives. Barbiturates and meprobamate have also been well documented as causing fixed drug eruptions in the mouth. The palate, lips or tongue are typical sites for the lesion to occur. On the palate and tongue it takes the form of an area of erythema which may be raised and painful. The lips usually form a crusted lesion. Evidence suggests that this type of lesion is produced by a delayed (Type IV) hypersensitivity reaction.

Oral Reactions to Other Drugs

Sodium phenytoin: This is a commonly used drug in the treatment of epilepsy. Gingival hyperplasia is a well-known reaction to this drug. Maximally the hyperplasia is seen to involve the interdental papilla. It is less marked in patients with good oral hygiene and absence of sub-gingival calculus. Edentulous patients cannot suffer from this condition.

Management of these cases from the oral point of view presents a difficult problem. If the mouth is kept clean and all calculi removed regularly the condition will be diminished, but this does not provide the whole answer. Sodium Phenytoin is such a useful drug in the control of severe epileptics that most neurologists are reluctant to make a change for the sake of the oral condition.

Salicylates: While it is rare for oral lesions to appear from systemic administration of salicylates, when aspirin is misused as a topical analgesic large aspirin burns can occur. Patients with toothache will often in desperation place an aspirin in the buccal sulcus by the offending tooth. A white marginal erosion can easily be produced, which if due to prolonged abuse will even have a raised hyperplastic edge.

A similar mucosal reaction may occur to chlormethiazole (Heminevrin) and emepronium (Cetiprin).

Cosmetic dermatitis of the lips: Considering the amount of cosmetics used this is an extremely rare condition. Usually there is a history of changing lipstick, but patients may suddenly become hypersensitive to their old lipstick after exposure to sunlight.

Reaction to acrylic dentures: Contrary to popular belief this is an extremely rare condition. Quite commonly patients get a very brisk erythematous reaction in the palate and mucosa of the alveolar ridges, after new dentures have been fitted. If the dentures have been incompletely heat cured there will still be free monomer in the acrylic. This is a highly irritant substance which is the cause of the reaction and it is often most pronounced where there is a large bulk of acrylic. In some cases the covered oral epithelium will become white, due to superficial necrosis.

Usually it is enough to soak the denture in water for a few days while the mouth is allowed to recover. If the condition persists it will be necessary to construct new dentures, but this time every effort should be made to ensure full polymerization.

Lichenoid eruptions to chlorpropamide, thiazides, methyldopa, gold, etc. are considered in Chapter 5 under lichen planus.

Mercury and lead poisoning: Strict industrial regulations have reduced the incidence of these diseases. Lead poisoning is by no means a dead condition. Apart from colicky abdominal pain, anaemia and neurological manifestations, oral lesions are characteristic by a blue line (Burtonian line) round the gingival margin. This is probably due to lead sulphide being deposited in the capillaries in the gingiva. Usually the gingivae are inflamed and bleed easily.

Only very small quantities of mercury are needed to cause poisoning. Mercury treatment for syphilis is a thing of the past, but there is still plenty of mercury used in industry and poisoning can occur from inhalation of the vapour. A tremor and peripheral neuropathy are the predominant neurological features, but again the gingivae bear the brunt of the oral onslaught, being red, hyperplastic and bleeding easily. There is even a tendency in chronic cases for the gingival condition to become so bad that teeth are exfoliated. A great deal of secondary infection occurs.

Bibliography

Halozenetis J. and Harley A. (1967) Uraemic stomatitis. *Oral Surg.* **23**, 573.
Jaspers M. T. (1975) Unusual oral lesions in a uremic patient. *Oral Surg.* **39**, 934.
Rook A., Wilkinson D. S. and Ebling F. J. G. (1968) *Textbook of Dermatology,* Vol. I and II. Oxford, Blackwell.
Shellow H. (1958) The mouth in certain diseases of the skin. *Am. J. Med. Sci.* **235**, 456.

Chapter 7

Oral and Facial Hyperpigmentation

Pigment Production

The normal pigment of skin and mucous membrane is due to melanin which is produced in the malanocyte. Tyrosine is converted into dihydroxyphenylalinine (DOPA) by the action of an enzyme containing copper. In turn DOPA is oxidized to melanin by the action of the enzyme dihydroxyphenlalinine oxidase (DOPA oxidase). Melanocytes are dendritic cells in the basal layer of skin or mucous membrane. By way of the dendrites the pigment is transported to malanophores where it is stored in the dermis.

In amphibia a polypeptide melanin stimulating hormone (MSH) can be isolated, which is produced by the anterior pituitary gland. Chemically this is very similar to ACTH which appears to have the same effect in humans, although there are claims made for a separate MSH which has never been isolated. Local factors may also cause the increase of melanin production, as seen after the exposure of the skin to sunlight.

Physiologically there may be an increase in pigmentation in pregnancy. In addition to increased pigmentation of areolar tissue of the breast, the genitalia and the abdomen (linea nigra in the midline of the abdomen) there may also be patchy pigmentation on the face and even the gingival tissue of the mouth.

Oral pigmentation is not necessarily of pathological significance. Fry and Almeyda (1968) report that pigmentation may be seen in the oral buccal mucosa, the mucosal aspect of the lips and gums, but rarely on the palate and tongue. This was seen in 38 per cent of people with coloured skins and 5 per cent of light-skinned people from Europe.

Increased Pigmentation of the Face

Freckles and moles

Both of these are too common to be regarded as a significant pathology. Freckles (ephelides) are pale brown macules which increase in size when exposed to the sun. They are more common in sandy haired children, tending to become less marked with increasing age. Non-hairy moles (lentigines) are dark brown macules which are not affected by the sun, but may increase in size during pregnancy, or even the endocrine changes of puberty. Some of these moles may be larger with a papular or even a verrucous appearance and may be hairy.

Pigmentation due to local irritation

It is natural for the skin to become darker with exposure to solar radiation, but drugs may make the skin photosensitive, e.g. the phenothiazine derivatives and tetracyclines. Xerodermia pigmentosa, porphyria cutanea tarda (South African porphyria) and pellagra are three rare conditions which cause the skin to react in an abnormal way to sunlight, which gives an inflammatory condition which will settle and eventually give increased pigmentation. Following radiotherapy there will be increased pigmentation with telangiectasia of small vessels in the skin. Skin appendages such as hair follicles, sebaceous glands and sweat glands tend to atrophy, giving the skin a smooth appearance with patchy pigmentation and vascular markings. Even exposure to heat can cause patchy pigmentation but this is more commonly seen on the legs and the abdomen (erythema ab igne).

A variety of chemical agents can cause pigmentation of the skin, the most common coming in contact with the face are essential oils in cosmetics, e.g. eau de Cologne, which may give pigmentation where it has been dabbed on to the skin. Tar workers often have hyperpigmented skin where they have been splashed; although this is more common on the arms, the face may be involved.

Any dermatosis which causes pruritus, scratching or picking of the skin can lead to pigmentation. Lichen planus is a good example of this but is by no means alone in the field.

Endocrine diseases causing excess pigmentation

Hyperactivity of the anterior pituitary with excess ACTH production can be associated with hyperpigmentation. This is more pronounced if there are defective suprarenal glands (Addison's disease) or if an adrenalectomy has been performed. Thyrotoxicosis may be associated with hyperpigmentation probably due to excess pituitary-like activity. Diabetes mellitus has been claimed to cause hyperpigmentation but the mechanism is not clear; the same must be said for the claims in hyperparathyroidism.

Albright's syndrome consists of the triad of fibrous dysplasia of bone, precocious sexual development, usually seen in females, and patchy pigmentation of the skin. It is not clear if the excess of oestrogens are responsible for the pigmentation.

Other diseases associated with hyperpigmentation

Neurofibromatosis may be associated with a café-au-lait pigmentation of the skin. The list of odd conditions that have pigmentation reported could be stretched indefinitely but let it suffice to say that tuberculosis, malaria, cirrhosis of the liver, malabsorption syndromes, xanthomatosis and even most long-standing diseases may be associated with pigmentation. Conditions that must be mentioned in slightly more detail are malignancy, haemochromatosis, haemosiderosis and the Peutz–Jegher's syndrome.

Malignancy: In some patients with metastatic malignancy there appears to be a polypeptide released by the tumour which is very similar to MSH, with the resultant diffuse pigmentation of the skin. This appears more localized in acanthosis nigricans, where there may be thickening and darkening of the skin in natural folds of the body. Acanthosis nigricans is not always associated with internal malignancy as there are juvenile forms which are quite benign and a pseudo acanthosis nigricans which may be associated with obesity. In the mouth it may not be pigmented and can easily be confused with a white spongy naevus.

Haemochromatosis: This is a rare condition where there are large quantities of iron pigments deposited in the skin; in the liver giving cirrhosis, in the pancreas giving diabetes, and even in the suprarenal glands giving suprarenal failure which may give added melanin pigmentation. In spite of the condition being called 'bronze diabetes' the skin is often a slate grey.

Haemosiderosis: This is a similar condition which has only been occurring since repeated transfusions have been given for haemolytic anaemia.

Peutz–Jegher's syndrome: This is a dominant familial condition in which there is the association of gastrointestinal polyposis and mucocutaneous pigmentation.

The intestinal polyps vary in size and number and may be situated anywhere in the alimentary tract. Usually the polyps are benign and cause obstruction of the alimentary tract that needs operation, but just under a quarter undergo malignant change. Melanomatous spots about 5 mm in diameter are seen around the lips in nearly every case and in the buccal mucosa in a high proportion of cases. There may even be pigmented spots around the eyes and nose, but more rarely on the trunk and extremities. Obviously these lesions have to be distinguished from freckles, which never occur in the mouth, and, finally, are not so darkly coloured. Pigmentation is rare at birth but appears soon after.

Diagnosis can be suspected by the distribution of pigmentation and can be confirmed by barium meal and follow-through or barium enema. A number of cases without a family history present with intestinal obstruction.

Malignant melanoma

Fortunately the majority of melanomas are benign but occasionally a mole may increase in size, bleed or ulcerate and there may be evidence of satellite melanoma round the periphery. This is a rapidly malignant tumour with metasteses to the regional lymph glands. Malignant changes are more commonly seen in melanoma under the nails and on the soles of feet or palms of hands. When this condition is suspected, a biopsy would only disseminate the condition, so a bold excision with a wide margin of tissue is the only hope. Occasionally metastatic melanoma give rise to melanin products in the urine (melanuria) which turns dark on standing.

Drug-induced pigmentation

There are a number of reports of meprobamate causing hyperpigmentation which persists for a long time after the drug has been withdrawn.

Some cytotoxic drugs also seem to have this property. Most of the heavy metals will cause pigmentation if injected. Hyperpigmentation has been reported in about 10 per cent of women taking oestrogens and progesterones continuously as a contraceptive.

Pigmentation of the oral mucosa

Compared with cutaneous pigmentation, oral mucosal pigmentation is less pronounced, but any of the conditions mentioned above, if they occur in a gross form, will give rise to oral pigmentation. The most common cause of oral pigmentation is idiopathic and it must be remembered that 5 per cent of light-skinned people have oral pigmentation. Occasionally young women who show a considerable amount of gum when they smile, become worried about increasing pigmentation of the gingiva.

At one time pigmentation of the oral mucosa was taken as being diagnostic of Addison's disease, but now it is well recognized as occurring in the Peutz–Jegher's syndrome, thyrotoxicosis, malabsorption and deficiency syndromes, cachetic states, disorders of iron metabolism and neurofibromatosis.

Fry and Almeyda (1968) suggest the following investigations to exclude endocrine and malabsorption disease:

1. Haemoglobin estimation.
2. Serum folate.
3. Xylose tolerance test.
4. Plasma cortisol estimations before and after ACTH stimulation.
5. Any other appropriate investigations according to clinical findings.

Heavy metal poisoning as seen on the gingiva

Poisoning with heavy metals such as mercury, bismuth and lead may produce a dark line just below the gingival margin. The suggestion is that soluble salts circulate in the blood and pass through the vessels of the gingiva, where they are exposed to sulphides due to bacterial action in the gingival pockets. Metallic sulphides are formed which become precipitated in the inflamed tissue, as there is always associated gingival inflammation.

Amalgam tattoo

This is extremely commonly found presenting as a dark bluish-black stain in an edentulous area of alveolus, where previously there was a tooth with heavy amalgam filling. Small particles of the amalgam become impregnated into the tissues to give a tattoo. This is distinct from a large piece of amalgam being left in the gum after extraction; the latter may require to be removed while the former needs no treatment.

Bibliography

Ellis H. (1967) The Peutz–Jegher's syndrome. *Hosp. Med.* **1,** 730.
Fry L. and Almeyda J. R. (1968) The incidence of buccal pigmentation in caucasoids and negroids in Britain. *Br. J. Dermatol.* **80,** 244.
Snell R. S. and Bischitz R. G. (1960) The effects of large doses of oestrogens and progesterones on melanin pigmentation. *J. Invest. Dermatol.* **35,** 73.
Staley C. J. and Schwarz H. (1957) Gastrointestinal polyposis and pigmentation of the oral mucosa (Peutz–Jegher's syndrome). *Int. Abst. Surg.* **105,** 1.

Chapter 8

Haemorrhagic and Vascular Lesions of the Oral Mucosa

Leukaemia

There is some variation in the oral condition according to the type of leukaemia. Acute leukaemias give more florid features, and the acute monoblastic leukaemia gives the most miserable oral features of them all. Modern methods of treatment, especially of acute leukaemias, has done much to alter the clinical features especially in the mouth. Fortunately, it is now not so common to see patients with gross oral lesions.

About 80 per cent of patients with acute monocytic leukaemia have some oral features. The most pronounced feature is swelling of the gums, which are stuffed full of leukaemic cells. Bleeding and gingival infection is common under these conditions. Large areas of tissue may become necrotic, leaving great ulcers. As can be imagined with this fearful state, the patient has great difficulty in eating and there is a most pronounced foetor ex ore. Death comes as a merciful end when the full severity of the condition is seen in the mouth.

Up to 50 per cent of other acute leukaemias have oral manifestations. If lymphadenopathy is included, then the percentage will be even higher. Gingival haemorrhage is the most common of the oral features, which occurs in about a quarter of cases. A slightly less frequent feature is ulcers of a non-specific type. About 5 per cent of patients have petechial haemorrhages or even frank areas of ecchymosis. The resistance of oral tissues is lowered, which gives place to the opportunist infections such as Vincent's infection and *Candida albicans*. Vincent's infection is so rare in children that all cases should be treated as suspected leukaemia until proved otherwise. These same infections are to be seen in acute monoblastic leukaemia. Facial palsy can rarely occur due to deposits of leukaemic tissue damaging the facial nerve.

Whereas acute leukaemias are more common in childhood, chronic leukaemias are seen in adults but may terminate in acute leukaemic states. Chronic lymphatic leukaemia is a disease not uncommonly seen in the elderly. Cases are seen which are so insidious that the patient dies of some other disease without the leukaemia appearing to affect their expectation of life. Oral manifestations occur in only about 12 per cent of patients with chronic leukaemia. Again, this is excluding lymphadenopathy. Many of the features are the same as acute leukaemia but not so severe.

Dental extraction is to be avoided in patients with acute leukaemia as the wound left often breaks down and forms the beginning of rather distressing oral lesions. In chronic leukaemias this does not seem to happen so often. Herpes zoster is a common condition to be superimposed on a chronic leukaemia. Herpes simplex of the secondary type is also common and runs a protracted course.

It is rare for oral lesions to be the primary lesion in chronic leukaemias, but in acute leukaemias this is not the case. Haematological investigation is advised in all children who present with oral lesions that cannot be readily accounted for. Bleeding following extraction may very occasionally be the primary manifestation.

Most leukaemias are associated with anaemia, but occasionally cases of chronic lymphatic leukaemia are seen with little in the way of anaemia. The majority of leukaemias can be diagnosed from the peripheral blood, but on some occasions it may be necessary to proceed to a marrow puncture to confirm the diagnosis.

Thrombocytopenia

When the platelet count falls below $150\,000\ c\ mm^{-3}$ the deficiency is known as thrombocytopenia, but spontaneous bleeding does not occur until the level has fallen below $10\,000\ c\ mm^{-3}$. Thrombocytopenia may be idiopathic, due to hypersensitivity or secondary to disease of the bone marrow. Hypersensitivity can occur due to the drug apronal (Sedormid); this has now been withdrawn from the market but quinine and quinidine may rarely produce thrombocytopenia. Marrow disease covers a wide range of conditions including leukaemia, aplastic anaemia or where the marrow has been invaded in multiple sites by neoplasm. Infections and collagen disease such as systemic lupus erythematosus may cause suppression of the bone marrow. Each can cause purpura, occasionally involving the mouth. Very rarely the number of platelets may be normal but they are defective, which is so in hereditary thrombocytopathic purpura (Glanzmann's disease). Haemorrhagic thrombocythaemia represents another very rare condition where the number of platelets may be increased but yet there may be haemorrhagic episodes.

All these conditions give rise to purpura. In about a third of cases there will be oral manifestations. Small areas of ecchymosis may be seen in the buccal mucosa and the lips. Purpuric spots may be seen in the oral mucosa, especially the soft palate and fauces. The gums bleed easily.

Coagulation Defects

Primary oral features are not a prominent part of coagulation defects. As far as the mouth is concerned they are more of surgical importance. Bleeding of the gums may be an early symptom.

Investigation of Haemorrhagic Conditions

The Hess test for capillary fragility is rarely of much help. This consists of applying a sphygmomanometer cuff to the arm inflated to half way between systolic and diastolic for five minutes and recording the number of purpuric spots produced. Haemoglobin and white cell count indicate if the haemorrhage has been prolonged or if there is an underlying leukaemia. A report is necessary on the platelets.

To prevent unreasonable laboratory requests, a report of platelets will be a useful screening test in all but cases that have frank haemorrhage. In these cases, or where platelets are reported as being sparse, a full platelet count must be demanded. Bleeding time (0–7 min, Duke) and clotting time (5–11 min, Lee and White) are only rough screening tests but are easily done as a clinical procedure.

Where a coagulation defect is suspected a prothrombin time (10–15 sec by the Quick one-stage technique) or even a thromboplastin generation time must be undertaken. The thromboplastin generation time is time-consuming for the laboratory and is done by a variety of techniques with varying results. More advanced techniques for the estimation of the various clotting factors may be needed in obscure cases. This will certainly be best advised by a haematologist and may need to be undertaken in a special centre.

Much effort can be saved in investigation by having an accurate history. This should include details of previous haemorrhagic episodes, drugs being taken, the occurrence of bruises, the way the patient has reacted to surgery and, last but not least, a family history.

Scurvy (Vitamin C) Deficiency

Although the exact function of ascorbic acid (vitamin C) is not known it has an important part to play in many vital metabolic systems. Mesenchymal tissue is dependent on adequate supplies of ascorbic acid. Even capillaries will break down in the deficiency syndrome of scurvy.

There are parts of Africa where the condition is endemic, but in most countries scurvy is only seen as a result of gross dietary deprivation but is commonly seen in the elderly in a subclinical form, according to recent surveys. Fresh fruit, which is an important source of vitamin C, is an item that for various reasons is often missing from the diet of elderly.

In Great Britain there are three groups of patients who suffer from scurvy: elderly men living alone, patients on long-term diets for peptic ulceration and 'food cranks' who live on very strange diets.

The classical clinical manifestations are perifollicular haemorrhages associated with hyperkeratotic hair follicles. Hairs in these situations have a 'cork-screw' appearance if they grow long enough, but normally they are brittle, breaking off giving a plucked chicken appearance. Areas of ecchymosis are common, especially on the calves, ankles and arms. There may be an anaemia which can be normochromic or macrocytic.

In the mouth features are variable. The most pronounced signs are seen in patients with poor oral hygiene and some teeth of their own. These patients have swollen, oedematous, bleeding gums which may even cover the teeth. Haemorrhage into these areas of gum will be seen, which may even be followed by large areas of necrosis. Not surprisingly, teeth may become loose and are even exfoliated. Patients who have their own teeth and good oral hygiene usually have less pronounced features in the mouth. Edentulous patients have very little in the way of oral features. Even in these cases there may be large haemorrhages into the palatal mucosa. Secondary infection, as with many oral conditions, is a prominent feature.

Diagnosis is generally made from clinical features but in doubtful or subchronic attacks a vitamin C estimation is useful. Urine estimations of ascorbic acid are easily done using the dye dichlorophenolindophenol, and form a useful screening test for clinical work. The normal patient excretes 10–60 mg of ascorbic acid in the urine per day. There are various saturation tests in which the patient is given a set dose orally each day and an estimate made of the number of days before excess is found in the urine. For research purposes the most accurate method of estimating leucocyte ascorbic acid is used. A differential diagnosis may be needed from haemorrhagic disease or leukaemia, but this can usually be differentiated by a blood film and specific tests for coagulation defects. It must be remembered that scurvy is in itself classified as a haemorrhagic disease causing increased capillary fragility. Thus the Hess test will be positive.

In any doubtful case little harm can be done by giving vitamin C in therapeutic doses of 200 mg tds, but a blood film is a wise precaution to exclude a leukaemia. A swab from the mouth will differentiate from Vincent's infection, which occasionally may appear haemorrhagic.

Hereditary Haemorrhagic Telangiectasia

Syn. Osler–Rendu–Weber syndrome.

This disease, inherited as a dominant, is not uncommon and presents as multiple small angiomas in the submucosa of the mouth, nose, pharynx and alimentary tract. Lesions may also occur on the skin of the face and fingers. They develop after puberty and increase in numbers thereafter. The angiomas are small, about 1–2 mm in size, with a slightly elevated smooth surface and are bright red. They lead to epistaxes and gastrointestinal bleeding and hence anaemia. The oral lesions may bleed; if they do they may be obliterated by touching with a diathermy.

Haemangiomas

The head and neck is the commonest site in the body for this hamartoma and the mouth is a frequent site.

Pathology

The basic pathological abnormality is a proliferation of endothelial cells which may form a solid mass though more usually a plexiform network of capillary-sized vessels is formed. In the majority of cases the vascular channels become grossly dilated, forming large blood-filled spaces with a sluggish blood flow.

On occasion a very dense fibrotic reaction develops between the vascular elements and this impacts more solidity to the lesion. Large haemangiomas may be connected to the vascular system by correspondingly large vessels. The vessels in haemangiomas, being abnormal, tend to bleed persistently as they do not show the normal contractile response to injury.

Clinical features

Most haemangiomas are noted at birth or in the first year but 15 per cent of cases develop in later years.

The lesions vary from a diffuse non-elevated lesion of the lamina propria of the mouth associated with corresponding naevus of the overlying skin. Much more commonly the abnormality is expressed as a substantial swelling which is soft and compressible. Larger tumours may cause extensive deformity but these are most unusual. The overlying

mucosa is normal except in the case of the tongue where some hypertrophy of papillae is not unusual. The lesions have a red or mauve hue. In
deep haemangiomas and those with much fibrosis the overlying mucosa
is of normal colour and the mass feels quite firm.

Sturge–Weber Syndrome

The Sturge–Weber syndrome of angioma of the meninges (which later
calcifies) and contralateral epilepsy associated with a cutaneous angioma
of the face which may, on occasion, be associated with an underlying
gingival angioma. This may be either simple staining of the mucosa or an
elevated lobular lesion.

Within cavernous haemangiomas may develop spherical concentric
calcifications termed phleboliths which may be mistaken for other
pathological calcifications.

Treatment

Many haemangiomas require no treatment but an unsightly swelling, or
one in which there is danger of trauma, may be treated by excision or by
injection of boiling water or sclerosing solution such as sodium
morrhuate or ethamoline. Quite exceptionally, cavernous haemangioma
occurs in the jaws, particularly the mandible. A radiolucency with abnormal bone pattern is noted and the jaw may be expanded. Tooth extraction may then be extremely hazardous. The aneurysmal bone cyst also
occurs in the mandible and is to be distinguished from haemangioma.
The subject is covered in texts of oral surgery.

Oral Phlebectasia

This has been well described by Rappaport and Shiffman. Varicosity of
the ranine veins is very common in the elderly and they describe small
localized venous pouches in the lips and cheeks of the elderly which they
call 'caviar spots'. This phlebectasia may be associated with scrotal and
jejunal phlebectasia—Fordyce's lesion. The jejunal phlebectasia may be
present as anaemia due to occult bleeding or with more urgent symptoms
of gastrointestinal haemorrhage.

Bibliography

Duffy J. H. and Driscoll E. J. (1958). Oral manifestations of leukaemia. *Oral Surg.* **11**,
    484.

Durocher R. T. et al. (1961) Oral manifestations of hereditary haemorrhagic telangectasia. *Oral Surg.* **14**, 550.

Lynch M. A. and Ship I. I. (1967) Internal oral manifestations of leukaemia. *J. Am. Dent. Assoc.* **75**, 932.

Peltier J. R. and Oliver R. M. (1961). Oral manifestations of idiopathic thrombocytopenic pupura. *Oral Surg.* **19**, 131.

Stafford J. L. (1965) Blood disease in relation to dentistry. *Ann. R. Coll. Surg. Engl.* **36**, 280.

Chapter 9

Diseases of the Tongue

There are several conditions unique to the tongue which require special consideration. They will be considered under the following headings:
1. Fissured tongue.
2. Scrotal tongue.
3. Geographical tongue.
4. Median rhomboid glossitis.
5. Ulceration of the tongue.
6. Depapillation of the tongue.
7. Black hairy tongue.
8. Sore tongue.

Fissured Tongue

This is a hereditary variant in which the dorsum of the tongue is slashed by deep (3–4 mm) irregular fissures about 1 cm in length. The sides of the fissures are devoid of papillae but otherwise the tongue is normally papillated. This appearance is of no significance. Occasionally a patient is seen complaining of a sore tongue which has this appearance. It is not known whether this soreness is specially related to the fissuring but it seems likely that the soreness should be considered and investigated as if the tongue were normal in appearance with the proviso that empirically anti-fungals may be helpful to the sore fissured tongue.

Scrotal Tongue (Lobulated tongue)

This is also a hereditary variant of normal. The dorsum of the tongue is divided by shallow interconnected depressions into lobules. The lobules themselves are clothed in normal papillated epithelium.

This appearance must be distinguished from the acquired lobulation of the tongue seen in the sicca (Sjögren's) syndrome which is very similar. The tongue shares with the rest of the mouth marked dryness in the sicca syndrome, and this normally allows simple distinction to be drawn between the two types of lobulation which can be confirmed by subsequent investigation.

Geographical Tongue (Erythema migrans linguae)

This is an unexplained condition in which a patch (or patches) of the tongue dorsum become depapillated. The patch(es) heal on one side and progress on the other so that they 'wander' over the tongue.

The lesions present as bald patches on the tongue with a slightly hyperkeratinized periphery which are occasionally sore. The patients should be reassured that the appearance is of no significance.

Median Rhomboid Glossitis

This is an acquired abnormality of unknown aetiology.

The epithelium is acanthotic, the surface keratotic (papillae are absent). The rete pegs are externally prolonged, the underlying connective tissue shows fibrosis and chronic inflammatory infiltrate.

Clinically the lesion presents an indurated diamond or rhomboid shaped patch of smooth or lobulated surface in the midline of the tongue just anterior to the circumvallate papillae.

It occurs in 0·1–0·2 per cent of tongues and is commoner in men, being rarely seen before middle age. Baughman (1971) has shown that the lesion is not apparent in children which makes a developmental aetiology unlikely.

The only importance of the lesion is to recognize it. It is asymptomatic.

Ulceration of the Tongue

a. Recurrent *aphthous* ulcers occur around the sides and on the ventral surface of the tongue.

b. The oral ulcers of *Behçet's* syndrome are seen on the dorsum of the tongue as well as on non-keratinized mucosa.

c. The oral lesions of *Reiter's* syndrome—patchy inflammation, miniature lesions akin to geographical tongue and ulcers are distributed as in Behçet's.

d. The lesions of pemphigus and pemphigoid tend not to affect the dorsum of the tongue but are common on the ventral surface.

e. The eruptions of *herpes simplex* affect all parts of the tongue while *zoster* of the mandibular division of the trigeminal is unilateral.

f. Mucous patches of *syphilis* affect the non-keratinized mucosa while the rare gummatous ulcer occurs in the midline of the dorsum.

g. *Tuberculous* ulcers are most commonly situated on the dorsum of the tongue.

h. Extensive erosive *lichen planus* may affect the dorsum of the tongue but the cheeks and attached gingivae are more prominently involved.

i. *Erythema multiforme* affects the sides of the tongue and ventral surface in common with other parts of the mobile oral mucosa more strikingly than the dorsum.

j. *Traumatic* ulceration of the tongue is rare. Exceptionally such an ulcer may persist for a long time in a patient with systemic problems such as heavy steroid therapy or diabetes.

k. *Neoplastic* ulceration of the tongue is seen most frequently on the lateral borders. It is the only cause of prolonged painless lingual ulceration.

Depapillation of the Tongue

Tongue papillae may be lost *locally* in association with geographical tongue or oral lichen planus. In the latter case they are replaced by rather homogeneous tessellated keratosis in the affected area.

Generalized loss of papillae is seen with iron, folate and vitamin-B_{12} deficiency and such tongues are usually, but not necessarily, sore. Depapillation in the deficiency states only affects the filiform papillae and the fungiform remain although they may become attenuated. Eventually the dorsal mucosa becomes extremely atrophic. Classically the iron-deficient tongue remains pale while the vitamin-B_{12} deficient tongue becomes red but that is by no means universal.

Similar appearances, which are rather rare in this country, may be produced by riboflavin and nicotinic-acid deficiency.

Black Hairy Tongue

In this condition an area of the dorsum (usually that affected by median rhomboid glossitis) develops extremely long filiform papillae which become stained brownish-black.

Aetiology and pathogenesis

Unknown. Although some overgrowth of pigment-producing organisms is assumed to cause the discoloration none have been demonstrated and the cause of the elongation of the papillae remains obscure.

Clinical features

The area involved is symmetrical about the midline of the tongue extending forward from the region of the circumvallate papillae. It may merge anteriorly and laterally with some normal mucosa but is commonly well demarcated. It is unique in appearance the only possibility of confusion being with the brown tongue which accompanies (and persists some while after) antibiotic therapy. In that condition however the papillae are not elongated but are all stained a light golden brown.

Treatment

Patients should be advised to scrape the patch (with a teaspoon) or brush it with a toothbrush to keep it under control. Occasionally after complete removal by curettage (under general anaesthesia) the lesion does not recur. Generally the patient accepts that he has to live with it once its benign nature is explained.

Sore Tongue

The complaint of a sore tongue, 'burning' in the tongue (which may be associated with similar symptoms in the lips and palate) is subdivisible into two groups:

a. Those with a visible abnormality;

b. Those without a visible abnormality.

Only (*b*) will be further considered. Although commonly no cause can be found it is essential to exclude iron, folate and vitamin-B_{12} deficiency. Any of these may produce a sore tongue without any visible abnormality. Diabetes is also said to have this effect but does so very rarely so testing for glycosuria is also required.

If, as is usual, all these tests are normal then the term 'glossodynia' is sometimes used to describe the remaining cases of unknown aetiology. Although the burning may be confined to the tongue it commonly affects the lips and palate as well. Most patients with this complaint are postmenopausal women (it never occurs in men) so it is tempting to attribute it to some hormonal factor, but the effect of hormones, such as oestrogens has not been tried.

The condition is for practical purposes untreatable but occasionally antidepressants are effective in abolishing the symptoms. Many of these patients attribute the onset of symptoms to the provision of a new set of dentures (allergy to acrylic). There has never however been unequivocal demonstration that this allergy occurs and if it did, it would be expected to produce mucosal changes.

Bibliography

Baughman R. A. (1971) Median rhomboid glossitis: a developmental anomaly? *Oral Surg.* **31,** 56.

Chapter 10

Granulomatous Conditions of the Oral Mucosa

Introduction

The lesions to be described here form swellings, either sessile or pedunculated, which arise from the lamina propria of the oral mucosa. The lesions have in common a pathological basis which is granulation tissue. In this chapter we shall consider:

1. Pyogenic granuloma.
2. Fibro-epithelial polyp.
3. Peripheral giant-cell granuloma.
4. Denture granuloma.
5. Foreign body granuloma.
6. Malignant granuloma.
7. Sarcoidosis.
8. Crohn's disease.
9. Histiocytosis-X.

The first three, pyogenic granuloma, fibro-epithelial polyp and peripheral giant-cell granuloma, are quite localized and benign. They are also common, as is the denture granuloma, while the rest of the lesions are very rare.

The word 'epulis' crops up frequently in connection with these common lesions, but literally translated it means 'upon the gum'. Thus it is not a diagnosis but an adjective describing position only. The pyogenic granuloma, fibro-epithelial polyp and peripheral giant-cell granuloma are the most common causes of epulides.

Pyogenic Granuloma (Granuloma pyogenicum)

These are epithelial-covered masses of granulation tissue arising without obvious source of irritation. They are most commonly seen in the mouth on the gum margin and adjacent alveolar mucosa, but may occur anywhere in the mouth, although they are rare on the palate. They also occur on the skin as 'proud flesh', on the fingers, the face and the nose.

Histopathology

The covering stratified squamous epithelium is usually thin and poorly keratinized; parakeratinization is usual.

The bulk of the lesion is composed of very vascular granulation tissue. The vessels are dilated and thin-walled and there are many solid endothelial buds. The stroma is of plump fibroblasts and much reticulin is seen. A great concentration of inflammatory cells is usual; polymorphonuclear leucocytes predominate, especially beneath areas of ulceration, but lymphocytes, plasma cells and macrophages are well represented. There may be areas of more mature fibrous tissue in the deeper parts, the base of the lesion being in the lamina propria.

Aetiology and pathogenesis

The aetiology is unknown, but it is most likely that there is an unnoticed small wound in which exuberant granulation tissue forms. Why this should persist relatively static for a long time, i.e. many months, is unknown. In the mouth pregnancy appears to be very commonly associated with pyogenic granuloma and it seems likely that the effects of large amounts of progesterone circulating in pregnancy predispose the oral mucosa to this exuberant response to minor trauma. The pyogenic granuloma cannot be distinguished clinically or pathologically from the exuberant gingival lesions termed the pregnancy tumour or epulis. The best term for these is the pyogenic granuloma of pregnancy.

Clinical features

At all sites (including the skin) this granuloma is a little more common in women, while considering oral lesions separately the greater importance of pregnancy is noted in that 75 per cent occur in women during the reproductive period, although no age is exempt.

Symptoms: Bleeding is the commonest symptom or alternatively the patient may note a lump in the mouth.

Signs: The pyogenic granuloma is seen as a faintly lobulated, dusky red lesion which bleeds to the touch. The surface may be ulcerated or partly covered with whitish slough if traumatized, but usually the surface is atrophic and shiny.

The most common site is the gingival margin. It is most important to distinguish it from the exuberant granulations which may occur around the mouth of a sinus in connection with a dead tooth, usually of the deciduous series.

Close examination of the adjacent tooth may reveal a possible source of local irritation, such as cervical caries, overhanging filling or parodontal pocket. In pregnancy the lesion is usually superimposed upon the widespread gingivitis common in the second and third trimesters. Detailed periodontal treatment and careful oral hygiene are vital in such cases.

Treatment

Excision under local anaesthesia is advised; if the lesion is at the gingival margin diathermy gingivoplasty should then be performed with the application of a gingival pack. Any local factors should receive attention at the same time.

During pregnancy excision is not advised, unless bleeding is particularly troublesome, as the lesion atrophies post-partum and may disappear completely or may evolve into a small residual fibro-epithelial polyp which can be readily excised.

Fibro-epithelial Polyp ('Fibroma')

This lesion is commonly seen in the mouth, usually on the gum margin, also in the cheek, lip or tongue. An identical lesion may be seen arising from the exposed vital pulp of the teeth of young people, when it is termed a pulp polyp. It is not a fibroma, though frequently referred to as such.

Histopathology

The surface is covered by mature stratified squamous epithelium. The basis of the lesion is fibrous tissue which is not encapsulated and merges imperceptibly with that of the lamina propria, from which the lesion arises. There may be a slight subepithelial infiltration of lymphocytes and plasma cells, but in a third of these lesions the fibrous tissue is quite cellular. Patchy dystrophic calcification may be seen in about a third of cases, and bone formation is not unusual.

Symptoms and signs

The patient usually complains of a lump, but frequently the lesion is noted on routing examination. This reveals a smooth, soft or firm, pink swelling either sessile or pedunculated. The surface may be slightly paler than the normal mucosa, due to hyperkeratinization. Alternatively a traumatic ulcer may be seen on the surface. The lesion clearly springs from the oral mucosa and the underlying tissue is not indurated. Regional lymphadenopathy is not a feature.

Treatment

Sessile lesions should be excised with an ellipse of adjacent mucosa which is undermined and sutured.

The much more common pedunculated lesions are excised through the base parallel with the mucosa and the raw area treated with Whitehead's varnish; if on the gingival margin a packing should be applied after appropriate gingivoplasty.

Histological examination is performed, as with all excised lesions.

Peripheral Giant-cell Granuloma (Giant-cell reparative granuloma, Osteoclastoma, Myeloid epulis)

Introduction

This lesion is peripheral in the sense that it arises from the lamina propria of the oral mucosa. This distinguishes it from the central giant-cell granuloma which arises within the maxilla or mandible.

The essential pathological tissue in both cases is identical and in histological specimens the origin can only be distinguished by noting the surrounding tissue, whether bone or mucosa. The abnormal tissue consists of vascular granulation tissue which is well interspersed with multinucleated giant cells. There is also histologically an identical appearance to the localized 'brown tumours' of hyperparathyroid bone disease, which occur in addition to diffuse osteoporosis and osteitis fibrosa. These brown tumours occur as locally destructive lesions which in the jaws are clinically and, as noted above, histologically identical to the central giant-cell granulomas.

The giant-cell granuloma as seen in the jaws thus occurs as part of an expression of overproduction of parathormone or as a purely localized lesion which is not associated with any metabolic disturbance or other skeletal abnormality.

In the absence of hyperparathyroid bone disease, the giant-cell granuloma is practically confined to the mandible or maxilla although localized, idiopathic lesions of identical histology have been noted very rarely in long bones.

Giant-cell lesions of the skeleton were at one time all called osteoclastomas and it was recognized that these varied from localized destructive masses to neoplasms with highly malignant qualities. With the characterization of these 'osteoclastomas' into different groups, it became recognized that giant-cell lesions which are now designated as osteoclastomas, or in the American literature as true giant-cell tumours of long bones, are almost never seen in the jaws.

Other giant-cell lesions of long bones, such as benign chondroblastoma and aneurysmal bone cyst are likewise exceedingly rare in the jaws.

Since the peripheral giant-cell granuloma has always followed the central jaw lesions, in nomenclature it was at first termed a peripheral osteoclastoma or, more non-committally, a giant-cell epulis.

When Jaffe introduced the term giant-cell reparative granuloma for central giant-cell jaw lesions, the peripheral lesion likewise acquired this name.

The word 'reparative' is, however, best omitted, as the endosseous lesion is purely destructive and there is no direct evidence that it or the peripheral type forms any part of a healing process.

Histopathology

The lesion is covered by thin stratified squamous epithelium which is poorly keratinized or parakeratinized, beneath which lies a narrow zone of fibrous tissue.

The bulk of the lesion consists of a mass of vascular granulation tissue through which the giant cells are distributed unevenly. These have 5–20 vacuolated nuclei with prominent nucleoli. Areas of haemorrhage and patchy fibrosis are common. Areas of osteoid (bone matrix) or woven bone are also common. Histochemically the giant cells resemble osteoclasts, but differ from foreign body giant cells in lacking non-specific esterase. The base of the lesion lies in the lamina propria.

Clinical features

The lesions are seen three times as often in women and occur in the 10–40 age group. They are more common in the maxilla.

Symptoms: The lesions present as a swelling or as bleeding from the mouth.

Signs: The lesion is seen to be a dusky red, lobulated fleshy mass moulded to the surface of adjacent teeth. Bleeding may be provoked by trauma, but not as readily as with pyogenic granuloma. Ulceration may also be seen. Clinically it is indistinguishable from the pyogenic granuloma. The lesion arises in the gingival margin or attached mucosa and is rarely seen away from the teeth, although it may be seen on the edentulous alveolar ridge. Large lesions may separate adjacent teeth.

X-rays often reveal no abnormality but may show irregular bone loss in the interseptal crest of bone. Very occasionally, what appears as a peripheral granuloma is seen by means of radiographs to be the small part of a central lesion.

Treatment

This is by surgical excision. If the lesion does not involve bone, it is simply excised, the gum being contoured and a gingival pack applied. With bone involvement the latter has to be curetted, smoothed and shaped and the area packed to allow healing by granulation.

Histological confirmation of the diagnosis of giant-cell granuloma of this nature should be followed by enquiry, and estimation of the serum calcium to exclude hyperparathyroidism. This latter is most rarely associated with peripheral (as opposed to central) giant-cell granuloma, but on occasion has led to the diagnosis.

Central giant-cell granuloma is indistinguishable on local clinical or histological examination from the brown tumour of hyperparathyroidism. Thus, every effort should be made to establish the diagnosis by biopsy, followed by exclusion of hyperparathyroidism, before local treatment of the jaw lesion. In the presence of that disease, no treatment need by directed to the jaw lesion, which remits spontaneously with proper management of the underlying metabolic lesion. The majority of cases of hyperparathyroidism can be excluded by the demonstration of a normal calcium and alkaline phosphatase on three separate occasions.

Denture Granuloma (Denture hyperplasia)

Histologically and in clinical appearance this lesion more closely resembles a fibro-epithelial polyp, but is clearly related to irritation from overextended denture flanges. No true granulomatous stage is observed, but the term denture granuloma is hallowed by long usage.

Pathogenesis

The lesion is clearly due to prolonged pressure on mobile tissues by a denture flange. It is seen only rarely with partial dentures. It appears to be related to two basic features, namely mobility of the denture and pressure from the flange.

Mobility is enhanced by ill-fitting dentures and in general is a feature of aged prosthetic appliances. It is greater in the edentulous lower jaw than in the upper, especially if the ridges are poor. Mobility is not a feature of partial dentures, and denture hyperplasia is unusual in association with partial prostheses.

The element of pressure is enhanced by overextension of denture flanges, by the perseverance of the patient and perhaps by low 'pain threshold'. Acquired overextension is frequently seen, due to progressive atrophy of the ridges.

Rather florid denture hyperplasia is not uncommon in Negroes.

The histopathological picture is of loose, relatively acellular fibrous tissue which is rather oedematous. The overlying mucosa shows keratinized or parakeratinized epithelium. There may be a slight infiltration of chronic inflammatory cells beneath the epithelium. At the junction of the lesion and normal mucosa ulceration may be seen and here dense mixed acute and chronic inflammatory cell infiltration is usual.

Clinical features

Due to the association with dentures, the lesion is seen in the elderly. It arises in the sulcus at the junction of the alveolar ridge and the surrounding mobile tissues; it is less common on the lingual than on the buccal side.

The lesions, being painless, are rarely noticed by the patient; they are usually diagnosed when the mouth is examined for new dentures.

The denture granuloma presents a smooth pink surface a little paler than normal mucosa. It lies parallel with the ridge and the base is clearly in the lamina propria and may be from 5 mm to over 3 cm long and about 5 to 10 mm high and a little less wide. Not uncommonly, two or three 'leaves' are present, the largest being closest to the ridge. In such a case the denture normally 'fits' with the flange occupying the space between the outer two leaves. The lesion has a soft elastic feel akin to a fibro-epithelial polyp. Regional lymphadenopathy is not a feature.

It is very important, in the assessment of such a case, especially if (as is usual) surgical treatment is contemplated, to consider the condition of the mouth with a view to enhancing the stability of the proposed new denture. One may consider the possibility of mylohyoid ridge reduction, sulcus deepening, epithelial inlays and the like.

Treatment

The treatment is surgical excision which may be performed under local analgesia in most cases (details are to be found in texts of oral surgery). The difficulty is to make a proper excision and maintain the depth of the sulcus. In the cases in which surgical treatment other than simple excision is contemplated, general anaethesia may be preferable.

Foreign Body Granuloma

On occasion, a small, tender, submucosal nodule forms in the mouth at the depths of the vestibule or beneath denture-bearing mucosa and on excision is seen to be a foreign body granuloma which is assumed to have arisen in response to material being forced through the mucosa in the act of chewing. Although most common in connection with edentulous areas, it may be seen in the mucosa related to the teeth.

Pathology

There are homogeneous areas of material which are surrounded by foreign body giant cells, lymphocytes, plasma cells, polymorphs and a surrounding fibrosis. In the edentulous the plaque may occur on the denture-bearing area and then superficial bone erosion may take place.

Clinical features

The lesion may draw attention to itself as a swelling but on occasion tenderness is a feature. In the cases of lesions beneath dentures it is common for the patient to find eating painful and examination reveals a plaque of thickened mucoperiosteum with considerable inflammation. At first it may be thought that denture trauma is the cause and the denture correspondingly is eased without relief before the true state of affairs becomes apparent. Such lesions should be excised in toto; if in an edentulous area a pack is sewn in to allow underlying granulation.

Rarely an acute abscess similar to a dental abscess occurs in a patient who is edentulous and radiographic examination fails to reveal a tooth root or cyst as the underlying cause. In such cases it is possible that foreign material is forced through the mucosa by the denture and the lesion heals with antibiotics.

Malignant Granuloma. (*Syn.* Wegener's granulomatosis, the lethal midline granuloma of the face)

This is a very rare group of diseases of unknown aetiology characterized by a fatal outcome. Clinically and pathologically, there is some doubt as to whether the group is homogeneous or should be further subdivided. At one end of the spectrum it appears to have some features of periarteritis nodosa and at the other, of a localized lymphosarcoma or reticulum-cell sarcoma with eroding rather than tumourous qualities. They will be considered as a homogeneous group, but reference will be made to the Wegener's type with extensive systemic involvement and the lethal midline granuloma type which is purely localized. There is growing conviction that these two types of disease are quite distinct and that the 'local' type is a variant of a malignant lymphoreticular neoplasm. In a number of such patients such a neoplasm may manifest itself.

Pathology and pathogenesis

The local lesion which occurs within and around the nose consists of granulation tissue with a very dense infiltrate of lymphocytes and plasma cells; giant cells are common and necrosis of the adjacent tissue is the rule. Vascular lesions typical of periarteritis nodosa, namely fibrinoid necrosis of the blood vessel walls with intimal proliferation and surrounding chronic inflammatory cell infiltration, are not uncommon.

In the Wegener's type similar granulomata may be seen throughout the respiratory tract, with widespread vascular lesions of the kidneys, muscles, nervous system and other organs occur. The aetiology is quite unknown but periarteritis nodosa has many features of an 'auto-immune' disease.

Clinical features

The disease appears to be much more common in men and mostly occurs before middle age. The lethal granuloma type is associated with nasal obstruction and epistaxes or may present as sinusitis. In the mouth there may be pain leading to extraction, following which characteristically the socket fails to heal. Later widespread necrosis with sequestration of associated bone with secondary infection lead to great suffering. Necrosis may extend to the skin of the face with terrible deformity. The patient remains surprisingly well with no evidence of systemic involvement except a raised ESR, but dies in up to six months from exhaustion or bronchopneumonia.

In the cases more akin to Wegener's granulomatosis there is often a history of prodromal minor nasal symptoms of rhinorrhoea, obstruction and pain, and then with the onset of the illness proper the patient develops a severe systemic illness with fever, malaise and there may be symptoms of pulmonary or renal disease. It is not uncommon for these patients to develop a florid hyperplastic gingivitis (with no specific histological features). The local nasal symptoms are as described above.

Nasal examination usually reveals mucosal inflammation; florid granulations may be present with polypi and crusting. Mucosal necrosis leads to ulceration. There may be some swelling noted in the mouth, but characteristically the lesion is either a socket which fails to heal or palatal ulceration followed by perforation.

Investigations are usually indicated by the nature of the symptoms and X-rays may indicate irregular bone destruction in the mouth, while the occipitomental reveals extensive soft-tissue swelling. Tomograms may be indicated to reveal the extent of facial bony necrosis.

Chest X-ray should be taken and in the Wegener's type rounded radiopacities are seen which represent granulomas similar to those of the nose.

Blood should be examined for anaemia, which is frequent, and measurement of the sedimentation rate, which is invariably raised due to hypergammaglobulinaemia. Repeated examination of the urine for albumin, red cells and casts is essential and the blood urea should be checked periodically.

The diagnosis is established with difficulty as the clinical features are of 'malignancy' but biopsy reveals granulation tissue only with extensive lymphocytic infiltration usually reported as 'no specific features'. The inexorable progress indicates the nature of affairs—but the problem is to obtain enough evidence early in the course of the disease to justify treatment.

Treatment

The 'local' type should be treated with radiotherapy while cases with Wegener's granulomatosis respond to steroids and cytotoxic therapy (usually azothiaprine), radiotherapy to the facial lesions not being usually necessary. The prognosis for the Wegener's group is not as bad as that of the 'local' type, death resulting from renal failure.

In view of the great rarity of the disease a strong case can be made out for collecting the patients together in one centre for treatment to establish the best regime.

Sarcoidosis

Introduction

This is a chronic disease of unknown aetiology with granulomatous lesions widespread in the body associated with a depression of certain immunological reactions. For some reason the alimentary tract, including the mouth, is relatively immune to the lesions of sarcoid.

Pathology and pathogenesis

The typical pathological lesion is a small epithelioid cell follicle, often with central giant cells but without caseation or tubercle bacilli (the non-caseating 'tubercle' follicle). The giant cells may contain crystalline asteroid bodies or, alternatively, spherical Schaumann bodies. In older lesions fibrosis develops. A similar pathological picture may be seen in association with infections due to fungi as well as mycobacteria and in beryllium or zirconium implantation. The immunological abnormalities typical of sarcoidosis are due to poor or absent cell-mediated (delayed hypersensitivity) reactions but whether these are of primary or secondary importance is not known. The disease is particularly common in Negroes and bears an enigmatic relationship to its histopathological cousin tuberculosis.

Clinical features

The commonest lesions of sarcoidosis in the head and neck are cervical lymphadenopathy, salivary and lacrimal gland enlargement and uveitis; the rarity of oral mucosal lesions is striking.

Mucosal lesions present as one or more firm submucosal nodules covered by normal mucosa. Such nodules are usually asymptomatic and are noted in patients with widespread systemic disease; only exceptionally does an oral lesion lead to discovery of the underlying disease. The true nature of the lesions is only revealed by histological examination.

Cervical lymphadenopathy is present in 80 per cent of cases of sarcoidosis and the parotid glands are enlarged in up to 6 per cent and in such cases xerostomia may occur.

In spite of the lack of clinical involvement, Cahn has shown that palatal biopsy in cases of sarcoidosis reveals typical features in 38 per cent of cases and Tillman has also obtained histological evidence of sarcoid from a gingival biopsy of clinically normal gum. Dawson-Watts has described a case with repeated gingival hyperplasia due to sarcoid tissue which probably represents a local sarcoid reaction to some irritant. A number of such cases have now been seen and an identical gingival lesion may occur with Crohn's disease. Whether such cases should be regarded as Crohn's disease or sarcoid localized to the mouth (local sarcoid reaction) is somewhat debatable.

Furthermore from time to time a case is seen with persistent enlarged, thickened, turgid and painful lip (usually the lower). This condition has been termed cheilitis granulomatosa (Meischer). Histologically the sarcoid-like picture is seen and detailed systemic investigation (for sarcoidosis) negative; this again must be regarded as a local sarcoid reaction.

Attempts have been made to relate this to the Melkersson–Rosenthal syndrome but in that the labial swelling is *transient* (angio-oedema). In some cases of this syndrome the repeated lip swelling, usually the upper, may lead to persistent rubbery enlargement of the lips which in some cases also has this histological appearance (the remainder are lymphoedematous). This confusion has probably been exacerbated by the well-known occurrence of sarcoidosis in the parotids with facial palsy (Heerfordt's uveoparotid syndrome).

In systemic disease where oral manifestations lead to the diagnosis the patient should be referred to an interested physician with certain essential investigations complete. These include chest X-ray and radiograph of the hands, an electrocardiogram, a serum calcium, plasma electrophoresis and ESR. The treatment of sarcoidosis is basically observation; use of steroids is indicated by certain specific criteria (uveitis and progressive pulmonary fibrosis).

Crohn's Disease (Regional ileitis)

This is a chronic granulomatous disease of the gut which most commonly affects the terminal ileum but has been noted from the anus to the mouth.

Aetiology and pathology

The aetiology is unknown but the clinical features suggest an unusual reaction to an extrinsic agent. Pathologically the damaged areas reveal dense infiltration with lymphocytes and plasma cells with sarcoid-like follicles of macrophage/lymphocytic aggregates and giant cells. As far as the oral mucosa is concerned the histology is identical to that seen in sarcoidosis and sarcoid-like reactions. The associated epithelium, oral or ileal, may be ulcerated.

Clinical features

Recurrent abdominal pain with diarrhoea is the main feature with radiological demonstration of thickening of the length of the gut wall at one or more sites. Oral ulceration may occur but may be related to malabsorption of iron, vitamin B_{12} or folate.

The disease affects young adults and is usually present for some years before diagnosis which may be made on the clinical and radiological features or at operation. A particular complication is the possibility of vitamin-B_{12} malabsorption. Pyoderma gangrenosum and erythema nodosum also occur.

The oral features (which are not common) include soft irregular swellings of the buccal sulcus which may be ulcerated. The axis of these lesions is along the vestibule and they are the colour of normal oral mucosa (they resemble small denture granulomas but of course are not related to the periphery of a denture).

In addition a bright red granulomatous hyperplasia involving the attached mucosa of the labial (maxillary or less commonly mandibular) alveolar process may be seen. This is indistinguishable from mucosal sarcoid-like lesion which is not associated with systemic involvement (*see above*).

It is unusual for oral lesions to occur without a long-standing history of gut disease (although that may have remained undiagnosed until involvement of the oral mucosa provided ready access to material for histological confirmation).

The first two cases reported with oral lesions were not confirmed 'at both ends' and so credit for the first complete report usually goes to Bishop et al. (1972), although Varley's case is better documented and there is reason to suppose that he recognized the significance of the oral features first.

Treatment

Intermittent courses of steroids may be used, or sulphasalazine, but many patients require excision or by-pass of the diseased gut (chronic postoperative fistulae are a common complication).

There is no specific treatment for the oral lesions (they are generally asymptomatic). Gross hyperplasia of attached mucosa may be reduced surgically and then kept in check with topical steroids (Adcortyl in Orabase).

Histiocytosis-X (Including the eosinophilic granuloma of bone, Hand–Schüller–Christian disease and Letterer–Siwe disease).

Definition

A disease characterized by a uniform pathological picture of proliferating histiocytes and eosinophilic leucocytes leading to areas of localized bone destruction or rarely widespread visceral infiltration. In spite of the uniform pathology the clinical picture is extremely varied, depending upon the distribution of the lesions and the rapidity of their progress.

Pathology

The cause of the disease is quite unknown. The pathological tissue consists of sheets of pale vacuolated histiocytes amongst which are scattered numbers of eosinophilic leucocytes. There is a loose vascular stroma to the lesion. Osseous lesions invariably occur but their distribution is variable although roughly correlated with age. Older children and adults have a few chronic (benign) lesions while in infants widespread visceral deposits occur in addition. The most malignant form seen in infants is often called the Letterer–Siwe disease; and the association of multiple osseous lesions, diabetes insipidus and exophthalmos Hand–Schüller–Christian disease, although there is such variation in the clinical picture that the use of such titles is confusing.

Clinical picture

At all ages the disease is commoner in males in the ratio of 3:1. The age of peak incidence is 3–5 years.

In infants the disease is characterized by failure to thrive and examination reveals hepatosplenomegaly, cutaneous infiltration, chronic otitis media (which may be bilateral) and low grade fever. There may be exophthalmos or diabetes insipidus and a skeletal survey reveals multiple osseous lesions. The prognosis is poor. In young children the lesions tend to be restricted to the skeleton and attention is drawn to them by pain and swelling. Oral manifestations are prominent in half of all the cases. In the jaws, bone destruction may lead to loosening and then exfoliation of teeth. Alternatively, teeth may be extracted in the belief that they are the cause of a dental abscess but the swelling persists and the socket fails to heal. Radiography of the jaw lesions reveals a radiolucent 'space-occupying' defect, the margins of which are fluffy or diffuse and the teeth or tooth germs in the area appear to be floating in space. Some sub-periosteal new bone formation is common but not invariable. Because of oral tenderness the oral hygiene may leave much to be desired with a corresponding deterioration in gingival condition which is compounded by an infiltration of pathological tissue.

Although the disease is rare in adults, osseous lesions may occur in the jaws as elsewhere. They are painful and radiography reveals much the same features as in children except that the lesion tends to be in the body of the jaw away from the teeth. It is to be distinguished from malignant disease of the jaw and an infected dental cyst.

Treatment

The clinical features of jaw lesions are sufficient to demand immediate exploration and the subsequent histological examination establishes the diagnosis. Then a skeletal radiographic survey is necessary to establish the presence of other lesions and in children investigations to exclude diabetes insipidus.

A solitary lesion thoroughly curetted at the time of operation may require no other treatment. Recurrent or disclosed lesions require deep X-ray therapy. Disseminated disease calls for steroids of cytotoxic drugs in full dosage.

Careful clinical and radiological follow-up is required.

Bibliography

Epulides

Bhaskar S. N. and Jacoway J. R. (1966) Peripheral fibroma and peripheral fibroma with calcification. *J. Am. Dent. Assoc.* **73**, 391.
Bhaskar S. N. and Jacoway J. R. (1966) Pyogenic granuloma—clinical features, incidence, histology and results of treatment. *J. Oral Surg.* **24**, 391.
Bullock W. K. and Luck J. V. (1957) Giant-cell tumour-like lesions of bone. *Calif. Med.* **87**, 32.
Cooke B. E. D. (1952) The fibrous epulis and the fibro-epithelial polyp: their histogenesis and natural history. *Br. Dent. J.* **93**, 305.
Jaffe H. L. (1953) Giant-cell reparative granuloma, traumatic bone cyst and fibrous (fibro-osseous) dysplasia of the jaw bones. *Oral Surg.* **6**, 159.
Kerr D. A. (1951) The granuloma pyogenicum. *Oral Surg.* **4**, 158.
Killey H. C. and Kay L. W. (1965) Giant-cell lesions of the jaws. *J. Int. Coll. Surg.* **44**, 262.

Lee K. W. (1968) The fibrous epulis and related lesions. *Periodontics* **6**, 277.

Malignant granuloma

Garrett J. R. and Ludman H. (1965) Delayed healing of an extraction socket caused by a malignant granulomatous condition. *Br. J. Oral Surg.* **3**, 92.

Harrison D. F. N. (1974) Non-healing granulomata of the upper respiratory tract. *Br. Med. J.* **2**, 205.

Mills C. P. (1967) Malignant granulomas and Wegener's granulomatosis. *Hosp. Med.* **2**, 183.

Sneddon I. B. (1963) The differential diagnosis of granulomata of the nose and throat. *Proc. R. Soc. Med.* **56**, 888.

Walton J. N. (1958) Giant-cell granulomas of the respiratory tract (Wegener's granulomatosis). *Br. Med. J.* **2**, 265.

Crohn's Disease

Bishop R. P. et al. (1972) Crohn's Disease of the mouth. *Gastroenterology* **62**, 302.

Croft C. B. and Wilkinson A. R. (1972) Ulceration of the mouth pharynx and larynx in Crohn's disease. *Br. J. Surg.* **59**, 249.

Crohn B. B. et al. (1932) Regional ileitis. *JAMA* **99**, 1323.

Dudeney T. P. (1969) Crohn's disease of the mouth. *Proc. R. Soc. Med.* **62**, 1237.

Eisenbud L. et al. (1972) Oral manifestations in Crohn's disease. *Oral Surg.* **34**, 770.

Issa M. (1971) Crohn's disease of the mouth. *Br. Dent. J.* **130**, 247.

Taylor V. E. and Smith C. J. (1975) Oral manifestations of Crohn's disease without demonstrable gastrointestinal lesions. *Oral Surg.* **39**, 58.

Varley E. W. B. (1972) Crohn's disease of the mouth. *Oral Surg.* **33**, 570.

Sarcoidosis

Cahn L., Blake M. N. and Stern D. (1964) Biopsies of normal appearing palates of patients with known sarcoidosis. *Oral Surg.* **18**, 342.

Dawson–Watts K. (1968) Sarcoid of the gingivae. *Br. J. Oral Surg.* **6**, 108.

Eisenbud L. et al (1971) Cheilitis granulomatosa. *Oral Surg.* **32**, 384.

Greenberg G., Anderson R., Sharpstone P. and Geraint–James D. (1964) Enlargement of the parotid gland due to sarcoidosis. *Br. Med. J.* **2**, 861.

Hamner J. E. and Schofield H. H. (1967) Cervical lymphadenopathy and parotid gland swelling in sarcoidosis *J. Am. Dent. Assoc.* **74**, 1224.

Laymon C. W. (1961) Cheilitis granulomatosa and Melkersson–Rosenthal syndrome. *Arch. Dermatol.* **83**, 112.

Orlean S. L. and O'Brien J. J. (1966) Sarcoidosis manifesting as a soft-tissue lesion in the floor of the mouth. *Oral Surg.* **21**, 819.

Tillman B. (1964) Sarcoidosis with unexpected oral manifestations. *Oral Surg.* **18**, 130.

Tillman B. (1966) Sarcoidosis of the tongue. *Oral Surg.* **21**, 190.

Histiocytosis-X

Blevins C., Dahlin D. C., Lovestedt S. A. and Kennedy R. L. J. (1959) Oral and dental manifestations of histiocytosis X. *Oral Surg.* **12**, 473.

Nelson W. E. (1964) *Textbook of Pediatrics*, Philadelphia, Saunders.

Shklar G., Taylor R. and Schwartz S. (1965) Oral lesions of eosinophilic granuloma. *Oral Surg.* **19**, 613.

Chapter 11

Tumours of the Mouth

These will be considered under the following main headings:

1. Primary Epithelial Neoplasms
   a. Papilloma and squamous-cell carcinoma
   b. Adenomas and adenocarcinomas ('salivary' tumours)
   c. Pigmented hamartomas and tumours

2. Primary Mesodermal Neoplasms
   a. Connective tissue tumours and sarcomas
   b. Lymphoid and reticular tumours

3. Metastatic Tumours
   Of all these tumours the commonest by far is the squamous-cell carcinoma and because in addition it carries a high mortality, it overshadows all the others in importance.

Papilloma and Squamous-cell Carcinoma

These tumours derive from the surface epithelium of the mouth.

Papilloma: The papilloma is rare; pathologically it is a localized hyperplasia of the surface epithelium usually well keratinized with a small core of connective tissue. Clinically, a papilloma is often asymptomatic and noted on routine examination. It usually occurs toward the back of the mouth on the fauces or soft palate or tongue. The appearance is diagnostic with a narrow pedicle and dilated head covered by white filiform projections, the overall size being up to 5 mm. Excision is the treatment of choice.

Squamous-cell Carcinoma: This accounts for at least 95 per cent of oral malignancies, and oral cancer deaths in Western countries comprise 5 per cent of all cancer deaths. The highest incidence of cancer is at the front of the mouth, on the lip, and is progressively less common to the

127

posterior, but conversely there is a tendency for anterior carcinomas to be less malignant than those derived from the posterior part of the tongue and fauces.

Aetiology

The aetiology of oral carcinoma is unknown but there are certain factors known to be associated with an increased incidence of this neoplasm, namely:
1. Sunlight.
2. Tobacco.
3. Alcohol.
4. Syphilis.
5. Candidosis.
6. Iron-deficiency anaemia.

Sunlight: This is only an important factor in the aetiology of carcinoma of the lip. It is thought to account for the increased incidence of the disease in the lower rather than the upper lip, and is particularly important in outdoor workers in sunny areas. The carcinogenic effect (which is shared by the exposed skin) does not apply to those endowed with a heavy melanin pigmentation of the skin.

Tobacco: This is the most important single identifiable aetiological agent. Tobacco may be smoked, chewed or placed in the mouth as snuff, and in each case may be carcinogenic to the oral mucosa. The smoking of cigarettes appears not to be associated with an increased incidence of oral cancer as opposed to its effect upon the upper and particularly the lower respiratory tract. Smoking of cigars and particularly pipes is associated with the form of palatine leucoplakia and hyperplasia of associated mucous glands known as stomatitis nicotinia. Although this is not itself precancerous, these habits predispose to carcinoma of the mouth, particularly the lip. In parts of India cigars are smoked with the lighted end in the mouth and this causes a high incidence of palatal cancer. In these cases the chemical action of tobacco is supplemented by the irritant effect of heat. When tobacco is placed in intimate contact with the oral epithelium it exerts its carcinogenic action which appears to be purely chemical. In parts of India tobacco is chewed with various other ingredients, including betel (areca) nut, lime and sandalwood, and this habit is a most important factor in oral cancer in India. For instance, in Bombay oral cancer accounts for 31 per cent of all cancer deaths while in Madras this percentage rises to 52 per cent. Although various factors such as malnutrition or heredity have been quoted as contributory, this is not borne out by the fact that amongst Madras inhabitants who do not chew tobacco the oral cancer deaths form 3 per cent of total cancer deaths, which is comparable to the European figure.

These 'chews' are habitually held in one part of the mouth and this area develops leucoplakia and then in 20 years or so a neoplasm, so that the habit is associated with carcinoma of the cheek, lower gingiva (alveolar mucosa), floor of the mouth and to a lesser extent the tongue. The constituent which is carcinogenic is not known for certain but is probably tobacco. For many years it has been thought to be the betel nut but this is chewed with lime, but not tobacco, among South Sea islanders who do not suffer an abnormally high incidence of oral cancer. In addition, the tobacco of certain districts (for instance, Manipuri) is associated with particularly high incidence of neoplasms.

Among Western communities tobacco is placed in the mouth in the habit known as 'snuff-dipping'. Snuff is powdered tobacco, often with spices, and snuff-dipping is a common practice among white women in the southern United States (Rosenfield and Callaway). This leads to the development of leucoplakia and in 20–30 years of cancer, usually of the cheek or lower alveolus. In the southern states of America such cancer is commoner in women than men (in general oral cancer is much more common in men than women) and in 90 per cent of patients is associated with 'snuff-dipping'.

In parenthesis, it is worth noting that nasal insufflation, the usual European method of indulging in snuff, does not appear to be an important factor in naso-antral carcinoma. In the Bantu race, however, who take snuff, naso-antral carcinoma is extremely common.

Alcohol: There is a close association between spirit drinking and carcinoma of the mouth in Europe and America: 51 per cent of the patients being heavy drinkers. There is, therefore, also a relationship between alcoholic cirrhosis of the liver and carcinoma of the mouth. Although the alcohol may have some direct action it seems much more likely that it acts indirectly, but the mechanism is unknown.

Syphilis: This is an important precursor of oral and especially lingual carcinoma. With the great reduction in tertiary syphilis and hence syphilitic glossitis, its overall importance is now much less than formerly, but syphilis should be specifically excluded in each case of oral carcinoma.

Candidosis: As has been mentioned elsewhere (Chapter 4), there is an association between speckled leucoplakia and hyperplastic candidosis and dyskeratosis in associated epithelium. It is unknown whether the candida plays any part in causing the dyskeratosis but it may be a potential cause.

Iron-deficiency anaemia: Severe iron deficiency in women may be associated with atrophy of oropharyngeal mucosae and dysphagia. In this Paterson–Brown–Kelly syndrome a hypopharyngeal web and later carcinoma may develop; also an increased incidence of oral cancer.

Oral sepsis and 'irritation from broken teeth' are mentioned only to be discarded. Although in many oral cancer patients the condition of the mouth often leaves much to be desired, it is no worse than a comparable control group. The teeth are usually carious with heavy deposits of calculus. Dentures, if worn, are commonly ancient and ill-fitting, but there is no evidence that irritation from teeth or dentures is important in the genesis of oral cancer.

Having considered the aetiological factors in oral carcinoma we shall now turn to the oral precancerous conditions.

Oral Precancerous Conditions

The implication of this term is a recognizable abnormality of the oral mucosa in which cancer develops more frequently than in normal mucosa. The problem is that the incidence of oral cancer in 'normal' epithelium is not known; for all we know all oral cancer may occur on visibly altered mucosa which is subsequently obscured by the growth of the neoplasm. It is in practice rare to see 'precancerous' lesions (including 'leucoplakia') in an oral cavity the seat of a squamous carcinoma. Some squamous carcinomas present as white lesions which are clinically indistinguishable from idiopathic or frictional keratosis. There is, however, much evidence to indicate that some lesions of the oral mucosa are precancerous as defined above. They include:

1. Chronic hyperplastic candidosis.
2. Sublingual 'butterfly' keratosis.
3. Tobacco-induced keratosis.
4. Idiopathic keratosis.
5. Syphilitic keratosis.
6. Lichen planus.
7. Oral submucous fibrosis.

As an addendum it must be noted that oral features may lead to the diagnosis of Gardner's, Peutz–Jegher's, Gorlin's, Cowden's syndromes; lingual neurofibromas/medullary carcinoma of the thyroid syndrome and acanthosis nigricans all of which may be associated with existing or subsequent carcinoma at *distant* sites. Their recognition is important in the prevention of such neoplasms.

Leucoplakia: The WHO definition of this condition is a white patch of the oral mucosa, which cannot be rubbed off and which is not due to an identifiable cause. The extreme weakness of this 'committee' definition is apparent, the major disadvantages being:

1. The more experienced the clinician, the more detailed the investigation, the more recognizable are the varying white patches. To the novitiate all white patches are 'leucoplakia'.

2. Histology is not considered—the majority of white patches of the oral mucosa are due to thickening/oedema of the epidermal layer of the oral mucosa and infiltration with chronic inflammatory cells. In some cases abnormalities of the epithelial cells in some way render the epithelium less transparent (more reflective).

The histology of such lesions may extend from:
1. Invasive squamous-cell carcinoma.
2. Carcinoma-in-situ.
3. Dyskeratosis.
4. Hyperkeratosis
5. Acanthosis $\left.\right\}$ multiple causes *see* Chapter 5.
6. Inflammatory changes

If histology were built into the definition then at least (1) and (2) of the above would not be included in the definition of leucoplakia, but of course it would carry the implication that all white patches should be biopsied.

Individually the precancerous lesions will now be considered.

1. *Chronic hyperplastic candidosis:* There appears to be an intimate relationship between this condition and subsequent carcinomas. When first seen the majority of such cases show dyskeratosis and a high proportion—perhaps almost 100 per cent—subsequently develop invasive squamous-cell carcinoma. The majority of such patients have no systemic disease accounting for the candidal mucosal lesion. Patients with recognizable immunological deficits etc. (*see* p. 62) seem not to develop subsequent oral carcinomas. There is a persisting debate as to whether the candida is primarily involved in the epithelial progress to

carcinoma, the alternative explanation (which at the moment seems more tenable) is that an epithelial dysplasia (aetiology unknown) occurs and the altered epithelium is less able to resist invasion of the opportunistic fungus. On this basis chronic hyperplastic candidosis (clinically recognizable but basically a histological entity) may require further subdivision.

2. *Sublingual 'butterfly' keratosis:* This is an easily recognizable lesion which is known to degenerate into invasive carcinoma in 50 per cent, often, however, many years after recognition.

3. *Tobacco-induced keratosis:* Stomatisis nicotinia (p. 76) appears not to be precancerous; the reason is not known.

Persistent pipe or cigarette smoking may induce keratotic changes in the lip which is precancerous.

Intra-orally, keratosis in heavy smokers (although commoner than in non-smokers) is associated with less subsequent carcinoma than that in non-smokers (idiopathic keratosis) (Einhorn and Wersall).

Period of observation	Tobacco users	White lesions in (17%) non-tobacco users
2 years	0·2	1·1
5 years	0·4	3·1

Cumulative incidence of carcinoma (%)

Similar figures are produced by Bánóczy and Sugár. Their figures relate to white patches in which tobacco, friction, alcohol, syphilis and candida played a possible role. With a mean period of observation of 8·7 years cancer was noted in 31 cases out of 520 patients (5·9 per cent).

They also noted the intimate relationship between 'erosive' leucoplakia (speckled leucoplakia) and subsequent carcinoma. No patient in their series with keratotic lesions only (leucoplakia simplex) developed carcinoma while in 82 'erosive' cases 23 carcinomas occurred.

It is hard to establish statistically a relationship between tobacco smoking and oral cancer. Perhaps tobacco smoking is only weakly carcinogenic to oral mucosa, or acts very slowly and so potential oral cancer patients die of other tobacco-related diseases too soon to allow evolution of the oral disease.

4. *Idiopathic keratosis:* When a white patch is noted with no identifiable cause it must be regarded with *caution* as subsequent carcinoma is more common than in many other white lesions (*see above*).

5. *Syphilitic keratosis:* This affects the dorsum of the tongue and is so rare (in this country) that syphilis cannot be counted a factor in the aetiology of oral carcinoma. It is indeed possible that the arsenic used in treatment was at one time an important aetiology (Binnie et al., 1972).

6. *Lichen planus:* This has long been thought not to carry with it the risk of development of cancer but in fact a steady trickle of cases of such association is seen in oral medicine clinics. Silverman and Griffith have shown that the incidence of carcinoma is 5 cases amongst 200 patients followed up for a variable period. Thus lichen planus must be regarded as at least as likely to malignant degeneration as 'leucoplakia'.

In all these cases the earliest clinical sign of the development of oral carcinoma is the occurrence of red shiny atrophic or velvety areas. Later of course more obvious clinical features occur with ulceration or papilliferous plaques.

7. *Oral submucous fibrosis:* This condition which affects 0·56 per cent of Indians is strongly associated with oral carcinoma which develops in about 25 per cent of cases. It is one of the small group of oral diseases that has no vulvovaginal counterpart. The tumours that develop in these cases are exophytic and of low-grade malignancy.

Pindborg suggests the oral submucous fibrosis predisposes the associated epithelium to the action of environmental carcinogens (of which chewed tobacco is prominent in India, *see above*).

Histology of precancerous lesions

Dyskeratosis (epithelial dysplasia, unquiet epithelium): This implies loss of the *regular* pattern of development of the cells from basal to surface layers. Abnormal cells are seen with increased mitosis—many away from the basal layer. Many of the changes are subtle and much experience of oral pathology is needed before these lesions can be assessed and the prognosis gauged.

Carcinoma-in-situ: This is simply an area of epithelium in which the normal cells have been replaced by others with the cytological features of neoplastic cells. It may be difficult to distinguish from dyskeratotic epithelium. Clinically carcinoma-in-situ may present as a white or red velvety plaque and the surface may be irregular or papilliferous. Such have occasionally been described as Bowen's disease or the erythroplasia of Queyrat. These eponymous titles are best avoided since Bowen described a roughened, pigmented, cutaneous plaque and Queyrat a red plaque of the glans penis, both of which are pathologically carcinoma-in-situ.

It is possible that invasive carcinoma develops from an area of carcinoma-in-situ, but the frequency of that change is not known. Treatment is usually surgical—wide excision and skin grafting are employed. Cryosurgery remains to be evaluated.

Squamous-cell Carcinoma

Pathogenesis and pathology

As noted above, squamous-cell carcinoma in the mouth frequently supervenes upon an area of abnormal epithelium but in spite of this and the accessibility of the mouth for examination, often develops to a large size before the patient presents for treatment.

Histologically the tumour is composed of sheets or clumps of eosinophilic cells, often with whorls of keratinization. According to the histological features the tumours may be graded from I to IV (Broders).

Among the least malignant lesions is a subgroup first named the verrucous carcinoma by Ackerman. In this, the neoplastic cells invade the lamina propria slightly but form a papilliferous mass on the surface. These tumours may be massive in surface area but it is unusual for them to involve adjacent bone and they do not metastasize.

The least malignant tumours tend to form papilliferous masses but with moderate spread into subadjacent tissues. The most malignant spread deeply, rather rapidly infiltrating through adjacent tissues with little surface involvement, which is noted as a deep necrotic ulcer. The majority lie between these extremes with a shallow necrotic centre, raised rolled edge and moderate infiltration. Apart from inexorable local spread, metastasis is via the lymphatics to the cervical lymph nodes. Haematogenous metastases occur late and although demonstrable in a large percentage of patients, at post-mortem they are seldom detected clinically nor do they materially contribute to the patient's demise.

Clinical features

Although early oral cancer may be detected as a small white or red plaque or small persistent fissure on the lip, the majority present as an exophytic papilliferous mass or an ulcer with greater or lesser induration and in almost every case there is no doubt as to the diagnosis. The patient usually presents because he has noted a swelling or bleeding: pain is unusual. The majority of patients are over 50 years on presentation and the disease is more common in men. On the lip the ratio is 10 male to 1 female but at all other sites is 3 male to 1 female (and falling). Most lesions are large at diagnosis and, except for the lip where 90 per cent are less than 2·0 cm in diameter when first seen, in all other sites 60 per cent are greater than 2·0 cm at that time. Lymph nodes are palpable in the neck in 20–50 per cent of patients except in connection with lip lesions when only 10 per cent have cervical lymphadenopathy. However, many of these lymph nodes are enlarged because of infection and the true significance of lymphadenopathy has to be assessed with this in mind.

The five-year survival rate is 85–90 per cent for the lip, and about 40–50 per cent for all other sites except the tongue in men, when it is only 20 per cent. Fortunately, the majority of oral cancers occur on the lip—between 25–30 per cent—but a further 20 per cent occur on the tongue, the remainder being distributed between the cheek, floor of mouth, gingiva and palate.

Management

If the diagnosis is suspected an immediate biopsy is mandatory. At the same time blood is taken for a haemoglobin and serology for syphilis. Careful radiological examination is essential to indicate local bone involvement.

Definitive treatment may be by surgery or radiotherapy but it is important that the patient is treated in a unit equipped to offer both types of treatment and to decide the best course in any individual case.

In general, surgery is preferred for small lesions and those on the lip; also for verrucous carcinomas and those invading bone. For larger lesions and anaplastic tumours radiotherapy is preferable and surgery is employed for those resistant to radiation, for recurrences and for removal of regional lymph nodes. The results of treatment are noted above.

Complications of radiotherapy

Radiotherapy which involves the mouth leads to certain inevitable sequelae, the effects of which may be mitigated by proper treatment planning at commencement of treatment.

In the first place there is a considerable reduction in salivary flow which is noted progressively after irradiation. This may cause dysphagia and difficulties with the retention of dentures and may play a large part in the aetiology of 'radiation' caries. The latter is a peculiar form of superficial leathery caries affecting the cervical margins of the teeth which develops within eighteen months of radiation. The most formidable complication is osteoradionecrosis of the mandible which is much less common now due to improved radiotherapeutic technique. It is due to progressive reduction in the blood supply of the mandible due to a progressive endarteritis. The bone becomes brittle but remains intact until exposed to infection by removal of a tooth or ulceration of a denture. The infection spreads within the bone causing widespread painful sequestration with a very prolonged course. In order to prevent osteoradionecrosis it is necessary to ensure that all carious, heavily filled and periodontally involved teeth are removed. A good rule is to have the mouth in such good condition that no extraction will be necessary in the succeeding five years. Frequently, a clearance is necessary and this is demanded by some authorities anyway.

Should tooth extraction be performed in a mandible which has been irradiated, it should be performed under antibiotic cover and this is continued till healing is complete. The extraction is performed atraumatically and the soft-tissue margins freshened and brought together to achieve soft-tissue cover for the socket.

Adenomas and Adenocarcinomas ('salivary' tumours)

Pathology: Salivary neoplasms fall into one of the following classes:

Epithelial:

1. Papillary cystadenoma lymphomatosum (Warthin's tumour).
2. Adenoma (pleomorphic).
3. Adenocarcinoma, including 'malignant pleomorphic adenoma'.
4. Adenocystic carcinoma.
5. Muco-epidermoid carcinoma.
6. Anaplastic carcinoma.

The pathology of these tumours is rather complicated and a textbook such as those of Lucas or Willis should be consulted. The papillary cystadenoma is entirely benign. The pleomorphic adenoma is normally benign but may be persistent and local recurrences occur. The remainder are malignant; the adenocystic and muco-epidermoid carcinomas tend to be locally aggressive tumours but may metastasize. The adenocarcinoma varies in malignancy but is generally very aggressive, as is the anaplastic carcinoma.

Parotid:

Clinical features

Of all salivary neoplasms the majority, over 80 per cent, occur in the parotid gland and among these the pleomorphic adenoma is most frequent, accounting for 65 per cent of parotid neoplasms. The papillary cystadenoma lymphomatosum is almost confined to the parotid gland but accounts for only 5 per cent of tumours here. The remaining one-third comprise the other varieties of epithelial tumours, all of which are malignant in varying degrees.

The papillary cystadenoma lymphomatosum is clinically distinct in that it occurs in elderly men. It forms a small, slight, mobile, firm swelling up to 1 cm in diameter which enlarges very slowly.

The common pleomorphic adenoma occurs more frequently in women and is seen at middle age and later. The patient complains of a swelling which enlarges progressively either quite rapidly or very slowly to form a faintly lobulated firm mass which may reach a large size. The swelling, which is not attached to the overlying skin, is painless and only slightly mobile. Regional lymph nodes are not enlarged. In the rare event of an adenoma arising in the deep portion of the gland, it presents in the mouth in the tonsillar fossa.

The malignant tumours tend to occur in a slightly older age group and are equally common among men and women. The growth of the tumour tends to be rapid (but length of history is no guide to pathology). Malignant tumours may be painful and definite but late indications of malignancy are involvement of the regional cervical lymph nodes, fixity to overlying skin, trismus, erosion of the ascending ramus of the mandible, as shown by radiographs, or facial nerve involvement.

Treatment

Papillary cystadenoma lymphomatosum may safely be left but enucleation may be performed. Superficial parotidectomy is the treatment of choice of adenomas. Carcinomas demand total parotidectomy. Anaplastic tumours may respond slightly to postoperative irradiation but this is not indicated for adenocystic or muco-epidermoid carcinomas. Prognosis for carcinomas is very poor.

Submandibular: In this gland there is an equal incidence of benign and malignant neoplasms and Warthin's tumour is never seen. The patient usually complains of a progressive swelling but this may be intermittent due to associated duct obstruction. As in the parotid, great difficulty may be experienced in distinguishing benign from malignant and again the features of the latter are pain, local fixation and involvement of regional lymph nodes.

Treatment

Excision of the gland is indicated for adenomas and small muco-epidermoid or adenocystic carcinomas. Anaplastic carcinomas or those extending beyond the gland require excision with *en bloc* dissection of the neck followed by irradiation.

Minor Glands (intra-oral): Tumours of the sublingual glands are rare; the sites of predilection in the mouth are the palate (mainly in the junction of the hard and soft palates), the upper lip and the retromolar pad, but may also occur in the tongue, cheek, lower lip and floor of mouth.

As in the submandibular gland, the incidence of benign and malignant tumours is about equal. Pleomorphic adenomas account for the benign tumours (papillary cystadenoma lymphomatosum almost never occurs in the mouth) and the majority of the carcinomas are adenocystic (cylindromas) while muco-epidermoid carcinomas are not uncommon. Other adenocarcinomas and anaplastic tumours are quite rare. Lesions of the upper lip are almost always pleomorphic adenomas, while the tongue has a high incidence of adenocystic carcinomas and in the retromolar fossa adenocarcinomas are not unusual.

The patient complains of a progressive swelling and examination reveals a firm, slightly mobile swelling covered by normal oral mucosa. Ulceration may occur with malignant tumours. Diagnosis is straightforward in the typical sites but care should be taken not to confuse malignant disease of the antrum with an essentially oral tumour.

Treatment

Excision biopsy of the smallest tumours is reasonable but in view of the uncertain nature of the histology biopsy is advisable for all tumours suspected of being salivary in origin. Pleomorphic adenomas are adequately treated by enucleation while adenocystic carcinomas, muco-epidermoids and adenocarcinomas require wide excision, and postoperative irradiation may be advised for the latter.

Pigmented Hamartomas and Tumours

These will be considered under the following headings:
1. Malignant melanomas.
2. Pigmented tumour of the jaws of infants.

Malignant Melanomas: These occur in the mouth; Calvera et al. were able to collect over 100 cases from the literature up to 1964. As is true of all melanotic tumours, they are exceedingly rare in those with extensive racial pigmentation.

The first sign is either a rapidly enlarging black mass in the mouth or progressive cervical lymphadenopathy. The primary is raised with a smooth surface and may fungate or ulcerate and the edge merges imperceptibly into surrounding tissue.

Treatment is by radiotherapy but the prognosis is very bad. Melanomas in the mouth may be metastatic.

Pigmented Tumour of the Jaws of Infants: This is a tumour which has many pseudonyms based largely upon theories of origin; hence the noncommittal title above. Synonyms include progonoma, retinal anlage tumour, melanotic ameloblastoma and pigmented epulis.

Pathology and pathogenesis

The origin of the tumour is unknown but it is thought to be derived from odontogenic tissue, although this obviously does not apply to the similar lesions occurring outside the jaws. There is a capsule enclosing an irregularly pigmented tumour. Histology reveals groups of epithelial cells and others containing pigment granules, the whole giving a decidedly bizarre and 'malignant' appearance belying the capsule.

Clinical features

The tumour may be present at birth and if not, is noted within the first six months of life. One or two similar tumours have been observed in adults. In 90 per cent of cases the midline of the maxilla is involved and attention is drawn to the tumour by swelling and its black or blue colour. It grows rapidly so that alarm may be generated, but the tumour is benign and treatment is surgical, the tumour being enucleated.

A similar tumour has been reported among this age group from sites outside the jaw.

Primary Mesodermal Neoplasms

Vascular Hamartomas and Tumours: The majority of vascular lesions in the mouth are developmental anomalies (hamartomas) rather than true neoplasms. They comprise one variety of naevus which term also embraces melanotic hamartomas (pigmented naevi) and the oral epithelial lesion of the white spongy naevus. The word thus has no pathological significance. The lesions to be considered here are:

1. Lymphangioma.
2. Angiosarcoma.

The vascular hamartomas are covered in Chapter 8.

Lymphangioma: This is much less common than haemangioma in the mouth. The vessels comprising the lesion are very thin-walled and contain no blood. Deep-seated, rather ill-defined haemangioma or lymphangioma may cause macrocheilia, usually of the upper lip, or macroglossia but in either case the cause is usually demonstrable since a small part of the tumour extends to the surface. Surgical treatment for these conditions may be indicated but may prove ineffective since total excision is not possible. Large cavernous lymphangioma of the neck is one of the common forms of the condition and requires surgical excision.

Angiosarcoma: This is a rare tumour of which there are several reported cases originating in the mouth. Histology reveals an anaplastic tumour with bizarre cell types but vessel formation may be noted. The tumour presents as a fleshy mass, often ulcerated, with a red or purple colour. The appearances are not diagnostic but biopsy is obviously required and indicates the diagnosis. Metastases are early and extensive and the prognosis grave. Treatment in the first instance is by radiotherapy.

Neural Tumours

These are *rare* and may be classified as neurilemmomas ('Schwannoma'), neurofibromas, multiple neurofibromatosis of von Recklinghausen and the malignant counterpart—the malignant 'Schwannoma'—which term avoids the use of 'sarcoma' and so the controversy of mesodermal or ectodermal origin is circumvented.

Neurilemmomas: These present as small firm nodules covered by normal oral mucosa, which grow slowly, occurring most frequently in the tongue. They are undistinguished clinically and, therefore, diagnosed after excision. Central neurilemmoma of the mandible accounts for about half of all such intra-osseous tumours in the body, which is undoubtedly due to the unique situation of the inferior dental nerve within bone.

The lesion may produce pain and paraesthesia or anaesthesia of the lower lip and reveals a central radiolucent area of the mandible which on close examination is seen to be a much expanded shadow of the inferior dental canal.

Again, the pathological nature becomes clear only after excision and histological examination.

Neurofibromas: These present as small soft nodules, submucosal, with no distinctive clinical features and may occur within the mandible. In von Recklinghausen's neurofibromatosis, cutaneous neurofibromas appear progressively until the patient may be quite covered by these small sessile or pedunculated soft lesions. This is associated with café-au-lait pigmentation (on the trunk) and occasionally skeletal deformities. Neurofibromas may also occur in the mouth and on occasion a large facial plexiform neurofibroma will cause extensive disfigurement. In this condition neurofibromas may occur within the mandible but are very rare in this situation. Malignant transformation occurs in the lesions in about 5 per cent of the neurofibromas in cases of von Recklinghausen's neurofibromatosis.

Multiple lingual neurofibromas may be noted in association with subsequent medullary carcinoma of the thyroid, their presence should initiate the search for the neoplasm; such an association is familial.

Granular-cell Myoblastoma (Abrikossoff's Tumour): This is a common oral tumour or hamartoma which occurs in infants and adults and has an unfortunate name since it is quite benign. Again there are many pseudonyms dependent upon theories of origin and despite their histological uniformity some authorities consider the lesions of neonates and adults to be distinct.

Pathology and pathogenesis

The pathological tissue lies beneath the epithelium and consists of an unencapsulated mass of large pale eosinophilic cells with small nuclei. In the neonatal type the overlying epithelium is somewhat atrophic but in adults is hyperplastic, sometimes to the extent of pseudo-epitheliomatous hyperplasia.

The tumour has been said to arise from striped muscle, fibroblasts or nervous tissue, but the majority view is for muscle. Willis is, however, of the view that the myoblastoma is degenerative rather than neoplastic, a view once held by Abrikossoff. The matter is sub judice.

Clinical features

In the neonate the tumour presents as a pedunculated or, more rarely, sessile swelling attached to the gum pad in the maxillary anterior region. The overlying mucosa looks normal.

In the adult the lesion forms a small plaque, slightly elevated, in the tongue, cheek or lip. The overlying mucosa may appear normal but more usually is white due to the epithelial hyperplasia and this may be the only clinical feature.

Treatment

Excision; recurrences do not occur.

Myomas: Benign muscle tumours in the mouth are excessively rare but both leiomyomas and rhabdomyomas have occurred. They form rounded masses growing in the tongue or cheek and are indistinguishable from fibromas, lipomas and deep haemangiomas. All such circumscribed swellings require excision and the tumour is then diagnosed histologically.

Myosarcomas: These are equally rare tumours of which a particular sub-group, the embryonal rhabdomyosarcoma, occurs particularly in the head and neck.

Pathology

The tumour is anaplastic with many mitoses. The typical cell is an eosinophilic granular cell but most of the tissue may be either round or spindle-celled and distinction from other sarcomas may be difficult.

Clinical features

The tumour develops in children often as a rapidly enlarging painless mass which may ulcerate. Diagnosis can only be effected by biopsy, there being no distinctive clinical features and treatment is by radiotherapy.

Lipomas: Benign tumours of adipose tissue are rare in the mouth as opposed to their common occurrence in subcutaneous sites on the trunk.

Pathology

The lipoma consists of an encapsulated mass of mature adipose tissue with a fibrous stroma.

Clinical features

The tumour occurs in adults, usually the elderly, and presents as a slowly enlarging mass. Usually close to the surface, its yellowish colour, with blood vessels stretched over the surface beneath the mucosa, indicates the nature of the tumour, which is very soft and elastic to the touch. Common sites are the tongue and floor of the mouth. Excision is the treatment of choice.

Fibromas: True fibromas of the mouth are exceedingly rare, the majority of fibrous overgrowths being obviously non-neoplastic.

Pathology

The tumour consists of a mass of fibrous tissue which may vary from extremely cellular to dense collagenous bundles with a few cells only. The cells are characteristically arranged in a whorled pattern.

Clinical features

These tumours usually form an expanding mass in the soft tissues though on occasion may be superficial and as it develops becomes pedunculated. The mucosa over the lesion is normal. Treatment is by excision.

Fibrosarcomas: These are rare; the histological features being similar to the fibroma, but the cells show malignant features with mitoses, enlarged nuclei and cellular pleomorphism. The clinical features are rather like the fibroma but expansion is more rapid and definitive treatment is excision and radiotherapy, but is somewhat disappointing.

Lymphoreticular Neoplasms

This group, although common, rarely present in the mouth as such, but as a cause of cervical lymphadenopathy they are mentioned in Chapter 20 and leukaemias are covered in Chapter 8.

Three are, however, of particular importance, namely Burkitt's tumour, plasma-cell tumours and the lymphocytic lymphoma of the hard/soft palate junction and they will be considered here.

Plasma-cell Tumours (Myeloma): These may be divided into three groups: soft-tissue myeloma, solitary (osseous) myeloma and multiple myelomatosis.

Pathology

These tumours are formed of neoplastic immature plasma cells which have a basophilic cytoplasm and large, eccentric, coarsely granulated nuclei.

Soft-tissue Myelomas: These are rare but occur particularly in connection with the upper respiratory tract. Usually solitary, they are treated by excision and radiotherapy but may develop into multiple myelomatosis. There is a form of hyperplastic gingivitis in which the excised tissue may be entirely filled with plasma cells but this probably does not represent a form of soft-tissue myeloma since myelomatosis does not occur. The exact nature and significance of plasma cell gingivitis is not known.

Solitary Myeloma: This has been reported as occurring in the jaws where it forms a painful swelling destroying the surrounding bone. Treatment is by curettage and radiotherapy but in many cases subsequently, sometimes after many years, myelomatosis ensues.

Multiple Myelomatosis: Deposits in the jaws are not uncommon in this condition and may draw attention to the disease by pain and swelling. Pathological fracture of the mandible may occur. Radiology reveals multiple osteolytic defects, particularly in the skull. It is a disease of the elderly affecting women more commonly than men. It may be diagnosed by demonstration of monoclonal hypergammaglobulinaemia (the sedimentation rate is grossly raised) with or without Bence–Jones proteinuria. Hypercalcaemia occurs and amyloidosis is a further complication. Treatment is by radiotherapy and cytotoxic drugs but the disease is universally fatal.

Burkitt's Tumour: This is a malignant multifocal lymphoid tumour of children occurring particularly in tropical Africa and corresponding areas of New Guinea and Brazil and rarely elsewhere.

Pathogenesis and pathology

The disease affects children of the age group 3–16 years particularly, and multiple simultaneous tumours develop. In the majority of cases the jaws are first affected but this is soon followed by evidence of neoplasms in abdominal organs, particularly the liver, kidney, spleen and ovaries. The lymph nodes are conspicuously spared. The tumours progress rapidly and death follows in up to one year.

The peculiar geographical limitation to humid, hot areas and below 1500 metres of altitude suggests that an insect vector transmitting a virus may be important in the aetiology. Reovirus and Epstein–Barr virus have been isolated from the neoplasm.

Histology of the lesions reveals a mass of cells like large lymphocytes with prominent nuclei with histiocytes dotted about containing abundant foamy cytoplasm and small dense nuclei.

Clinical features

The child presents with swelling of the jaw, more often the maxilla. The tumour originates within the bone and enlarges rapidly, destroying bone and causing deformity with loosening, then exfoliation, of the associated teeth. More than one tumour is commonly present in the mouth and all four quadrants may be involved. There is no pain and the tumours are not tender. Radiographically the earliest sign is an area of osteolysis in connection with the germs of developing teeth. Later there is extensive osteolysis, the teeth apparently floating in space. Involvement of the abdomen is revealed by swelling and examination reveals the organ or organs involved. Lymph nodes are not enlarged and there are *no* characteristic haematological findings. Treatment is by means of either methotrexate, cyclophosphamide or vincristine. The effect of radiotherapy is unknown but is less likely to be effective in a multicentric tumour.

Rapid remission is usual but recrudescence occurs and the overall mortality is high. When remission occurs it is probably due to the development of host immunity.

Lymphocytic Lymphoma of the Palate: This, as described by Tomich and Shafer, appears to be an entity. The lesion occurs in the elderly (70 yrs) as a soft mass at the hard/soft palate junction. Histologically the lesions are lymphocytic lymphomas. Dissemination occurs in at least 50 per cent of cases so chemotherapy or radiotherapy is indicated. It is important to distinguish this disorder from florid Sjögren's disease lesions which may occur at this site.

Metastatic Tumours

Oral metastases derived from neoplasms outside the mouth are unusual and it is exceptional for an occult malignancy to be diagnosed on the basis of an oral lesion. The primary is usually a carcinoma but may be a sarcoma.

Pathology

The metastases clearly spread to the mouth via the bloodstream and derive from many sites but particularly the bronchus, breast, kidney, large bowel, prostate and thyroid. If these tumours invade the jaws, they usually produce bone destruction with no periosteal reaction. If teeth are involved they may be resorbed but usually progress is so rapid that the teeth are left undamaged, the surrounding bone being removed piecemeal. Occasionally osteoblastic metastases occur, the malignant cells infiltrating the jaw stimulating the adjacent osteoblasts to produce new bone. Such neoplasms derive from the breast or prostate.

Clinical features

Deposits may develop in the soft tissue of the mouth, often in the gingival margin where rapid proliferation leads to the development of a maroon fleshy mass. This may be indistinguishable from the peripheral giant-cell granuloma and diagnosis is revealed only by histological examination. Many such gingival metastases derive from renal carcinoma. In the majority of cases oral metastases occur in the jaws, particularly the mandible, where they commonly lodge in relationship to the inferior dental canal at the angle of the mandible. Pain may be the first symptom but is rapidly succeeded by swelling and paraesthesia or anaesthesia of the mental nerve. Alternatively, pathological fracture may occur. Radiographs reveal a roughly circular area of bone destruction with very irregular fluffy edges. A similar clinical picture may occur with central adenocarcinoma, myeloma and sarcomas or histiocytosis-X. A tumour in the alveolus of the jaw commonly presents as a rapidly expanding swelling which looks inflammatory and is treated by tooth extraction. Subsequently, the tumour fungates from the tooth socket: radiographs reveal bone destruction and biopsy the diagnosis.

All such patients require admission for investigation and management of the underlying disease. Occasionally local treatment in the shape of radiotherapy is indicated.

Bibliography

Ackerman L. V. (1948) Verrucous carcinoma of the oral cavity. *Surgery* **23**, 670.
Bánóczy J. and Sugár L. (1972) Longitudinal studies in oral leukoplakias. *J. Oral Pathol.* **1**, 265.
Binnie W. H., Cawson R. A., Hill G. B. and Soaper A. E. (1972) *Oral Cancer in England and Wales*. London, HMSO.
Bling H. E. and Wagner J. E. (1964) Aneurysmal bone cysts of the mandible. *Oral Surg.* **18**, 646.
Cabrera A., de la Pava S. and Pickren J. W. (1964) Primary malignant melanona of the oral cavity. *Oral Surg.* **18**, 77.
Cawson R. A. (1969) Leukoplakia and oral cancer. *Proc. R. Soc. Med.* **62**, 610.
Coffin F. (1964) Cancer and the dental surgeon. *Br. Dent. J.* **116**, 191, 243.
Csiba A. (1967) A buccal lipoma of unusual size. *Oral Surg.* **24**, 527.
Einhorn J. and Wersäll J. (1967) Incidence of oral carcinoma in patients with leucoplakia of the oral mucosa. *Cancer* **20**, 2189.
Eisen M. J. (1946) Betel chewing among natives of South-West Pacific islands—lack of carcinogenic action. *Cancer Res.* **6**, 139.
Eversole L. R. (1969) Central benign and malignant neural neoplasms of the jaws—a review. *J. Oral Surg.* **27**, 716.
Fonts E. A., Greenlaw R. H., Rush B. F. and Rovin S. (1969) Verrucous squamous cell carcinoma of the oral cavity. *Cancer* **23**, 152.
Hagy D. M., Halperin V. and Wood C. iii (1964) Leiomyoma of the oral cavity. *Oral Surg.* **17**, 748.
Halozenetis J. Q. and Asprides H. (1967) Neurilemmoma (Schwannoma) of the oral cavity. *Oral Surg.* **24**, 510.
Hammond H. L. and Calderwood R. B. (1969) Malignant peripheral nerve sheath tumours of the oral cavity. *Oral Surg.* **28**, 97.
Harrison D. F. N. (1964) Snuff and cancer of the nasopharynx *Br. Med. J.* **2**, 1649.
Horton J. E. (1968) Lipomas of the tongue. *Oral Surg.* **25**, 914.
Kerr D. A. and Pullon P. A. (1964) A study of the pigmented tumours of the jaws of infants. *Oral Surg.* **18**, 759.
King O. H., Blankenship J. P., King W. A. and Coleman S. A. (1967) The frequency of pigmented naevi in the oral cavity. *Oral Surg.* **23**, 82.
Khanolkar V. R. (1944) Oral cancer in Bombay, India. *Cancer Res.* **4**, 313.
Kramer I. R. H. (1969) Precancerous conditions of the oral mucosa. *Ann. R. Coll. Surg.* **45**, 340.
Lemmon F. R., Walden R. T. and Woods R. W. (1964) Cancer of the lung and mouth in Seventh Day Adventists. *Cancer* **17**, 486.
Lucas R. B. (1964) *Pathology of Tumours of the Oral Tissues*, London, Churchill.
MacDonald D. G. (1969) Smooth muscle tumours of the mouth *Br. J. Oral Surg.* **6**, 207.
Macgregor A. J. and Dyson D. P. (1966) Oral lipoma. *Oral Surg.* **21**, 770.
Mack L. M. and Woodward H. W. (1968) Blue naevus of the oral mucous membrane. *Oral Surg.* **25**, 929.

148   CLINICAL ORAL MEDICINE

Mark H. I. and Kaplan S. I. (1967) 'Blue naevus of the oral cavity—a review.' *Oral Surg.* **24,** 151.

Mincer H. H. et al. (1972) Observations on the clinical characteristics of oral lesions showing histologic epithelial dysplasia. *Oral Surg.* **33,** 389.

Murray–Walker D. (1973) Oral mucosal nuroma-medullary thyroid carcinoma syndrome. *Br. J. Dermatol.* **88,** 599.

O'Day R. A., Soule E. H. and Gores R. J. (1965) Embryonal rhabdomyosarcoma of the oral soft tissues. *Oral Surg.* **20,** 85.

Omar–Ahmad J. S. M. and Ramanathan K. (1968) Oral carcinoma; a review of the aetiological factors and a preventive programme. *Med. J. of Malaya* **22,** 172.

Pindborg J. J. (1972) Is submucous fibrosis a precancerous condition in the oral cavity? *Int. Dent. J.* **22,** 474.

Pindborg J. J., Kiaer J. and Gupta P. C. (1967) Studies in oral leukoplakia. *Bull. WHO* **37,** 109.

Pindborg J. J. and Sirsat S. M. (1966) Oral submucous fibrosis. *Oral Surg.* **22,** 764.

Rappaport I. and Shiffman M. A. (1964) The significance of oral angiomas. *Oral Surg.* **17,** 263.

Shafer W. G. (1975) Oral carcinoma in situ. *Oral Surg.* **39,** 227.

Shklar G. and Meyer I. (1965) Vascular tumours of the mouth and jaws. *Oral Surg.* **19,** 335.

Tuyns A. J. and Hirayama J. (1966) Epidemiological studies of tumours of the mouth and jaws. *J. Dent. Res.* **45,** 535.

Wahi P. N. (1968) The epidemiology of oral and oropharyngeal cancer. *Bull. WHO* **38,** 495.

Williams E. D. and Pollock D. J. (1966) Multiple mucosal neuromata with endocrine tumours: a syndrome allied to von Recklinghausen's disease. *S. Pathol. Bact.* **91,** 71.

Williamson J. J. (1964) Erythroplasia of Queyrat of the buccal mucous membrane. *Oral Surg.* **17,** 308.

Willis R. A. (1967) *The pathology of tumours,* 4th ed. London, Butterworth.

Lymphorecticular neoplasms

Adatia A. K. (1964) Dental tissues and Burkitt's tumour. *Oral Surg.* **25,** 221.

Burkitt D. (1966) Malignant lymphoma of the jaws. *J. Dent. Res.* **45,** 554.

Cataldo E. and Meyer I. (1966) Solitary and multiple plasma cell tumours of the jaws and oral cavity. *Oral Surg.* **22,** 628.

Henderson D. and Rowe N. L. (1969) Myelomatosis affecting the jaws. *Br. J. Oral Surg.* **6,** 161.

Poswillo D. (1968) Plasmacytosis of the gingiva. *Br. J. Oral Surg.* **5,** 194.

Tomich C. E. and Shafer W. G. (1975) Lymphoproliferative disease of the hard palate: A clinico-pathologic entity. *Oral Surg.* **39,** 754.

Metastatic tumours

Cash C. D., Royer R. Q. and Dahlin D. C. S. (1961) Metastatic tumours of the jaws. *Oral Surg.* **14,** 897.

Cawson R. A. (1959) Secondary carcinoma of the mandible. *Dental Pract.* **9,** 240.

Cohen B. (1958) Secondary tumours of the mandible. *Ann. R. Coll. Surg.* **23,** 118.

Robinson R. E. and Stuteville O. H. (1962) Metastatic tumours of the tongue. *Oral Surg.* **15,** 980.

Salman I. and Lange I. (1954) Metastatic tumours of the oral cavity. *Oral Surg.* **7,** 1141.

Chapter 12

Diseases of the Salivary Glands

In this chapter the diseases of the salivary glands will be considered; ptyalism and xerostomia will be discussed separately.

The material will be arranged in a rather unorthodox way: by clinical presentation.

1. *Acute Swellings*
a. Mumps.
b. Acute bacterial parotitis.
c. Acute submandibular sialadenitis.

2. *Persistent or Recurrent Swellings*
a. Essential parotidomegaly.
b. Work hypertrophy.
c. Malnutrition.
d. Drugs.
e. Recurrent parotid sialadenitis.
f. Recurrent submandibular sialadenitis.
g. Sicca syndrome (Sjögren's syndrome and Mikulicz's disease).

3. *Localized Mass in Salivary Glands*
a. Inflammatory.
b. Neoplastic.

4. *The Mucocoele*

Acute Swellings

Mumps (epidemic parotitis): This is a viral disease which is quite infective and so predominantly affects children. The incubation period is 14–21 days and an attack generally confers lifelong immunity.

Clinical features

There may be a short non-specific prodromal illness and the presentation is a bilateral parotitis in two-thirds of cases. There may be a day or two between

149

the involvement of the second parotid gland. In the remaining one-third of cases, the parotitis is unilateral. In only 1 per cent of cases is the parotid *not* involved.

The parotid swelling develops rapidly and is painful, causing trismus. The orifice of the parotid duct is inflamed. Palpation reveals a smooth, firm, tender swelling retaining a typical parotid outline and there is overlying oedema.

The submandibular glands are involved in about 13 per cent of cases and bilateral involvement occurs in 5 per cent of cases. Submandibular gland involvement, the parotid spared, is exceptional, occurring in only 1 per cent of cases (as noted above).

Submandibular gland involvement is associated with overlying oedema and this may extend as presternal oedema.

The salivary gland swelling persists for about one week, occasionally longer. Suppuration never occurs. Extra salivary manifestations are much more common in adults and tend to develop 4–5 days after parotitis, although they may precede it or be delayed for up to three weeks. The most common manifestation is epididymo-orchitis (25 per cent of adult males). Meningo-encephalitis occurs in 2–5 per cent and is the most formidable complication, although complete resolution is the rule. Pancreatitis occurs in a very small number of cases and acute appendicitis only rarely. Transient myocarditis may develop.

Testicular atrophy is the only permanent sequel, and this only exceptionally following the most acute cases of orchitis.

The relationship between mumps and later chronic recurrent parotitis or submandibular sialadenitis is often debated. It can, however, play little direct part in the aetiology of an unusual disorder of adults, occurring as it does almost universally in childhood.

Diagnosis is usually straightforward on clinical grounds, but in difficult or doubtful cases (usually among adults) estimation of antibodies to S+V antigens and a complement-fixation test may help retrospectively. More immediately, serum amylase is invariably raised in mumps.

Acute Bacterial Parotitis: This is an ascending infection and is usually seen in debilitated and dehydrated patients. Once common in patients after abdominal operations, it is now a rarity, being usually seen as a rare event in chronic recurrent parotitis, but even there it is not as common as one would expect.

It presents as an acute unilateral parotid swelling with severe pain and trismus. High fever and leucocytosis are the rule.

The principal difficulty in diagnosis, apart from mumps in the early stages, is acute submasseteric abscess. Clinically the two may be almost indistinguishable and the distinction between them is made on the preceding history and the presence or absence of secretion in the corresponding parotid duct.

Treatment consists of rehydration, where necessary, and antibiotics; drainage is indicated in the absence of early relief. As the infection is most commonly due to *Staphylococcus aureus* and is thus likely to be resistant to penicillin, either methicillin or cloxacillin is indicated.

Acute Submandibular Sialadenitis: This is quite rare in comparison with local lymphadenitis and submandibular space infection. It develops in cases of calculous obstruction of the submandibular duct. Antibiotics are the treatment of choice and incision may be necessary.

Persistent or Recurrent Salivary Swellings (Parotid)

- *a.* 'Essential' parotidomegaly.
- *b.* Work hypertrophy.
- *c.* Malnutrition.
- *d.* Drugs.
- *e.* Recurrent parotid sialadenitis.
- *f.* Recurrent submandibular sialadenitis.
- *g.* Sicca syndrome: Sjögren's syndrome, Mikulicz's disease, benign lympho-epithelial lesion.

'Essential' Parotidomegaly: The name applied by Maynard to the symmetrical parotid enlargement in middle-aged or elderly men due to fatty infiltration. The swelling is painless and does not progress beyond moderate increase in size of the glands.

Work Hypertrophy: Seen but rarely in people of curious dietary habits involving a large intake of starch.

Malnutrition: Associated with persistent symmetrical, painless parotidomegaly and is most frequently seen in this country in alcoholics. It is, therefore, associated with alcoholic cirrhosis of the liver. Such parotidomegaly has also been seen in starving people, including prisoners of war, and remits upon improvement of the nutritional standard of the patient.

Drugs: Have been noted as a cause of parotid swelling which may be either acute (and closely resemble mumps) or chronic. The acute cases may be associated with other hypersensitivity phenomena and are themselves considered to be allergic in character. The submandibular gland may be swollen also. The drug most frequently responsible is phenylbutazone.

Many drugs produce dryness of the mouth as a side effect and guanethidine produces parotid pain without swelling. Bruce-Pearson has described cases of recurrent parotid enlargement in which allergy appears to be of prime importance and these cases are associated with diminished parotid salivary flow. The viscid secretion, if examined, contains many eosinophils and in all the cases a marked blood eosinophilia is present. Bruce-Pearson considers such cases to account for 15 per cent of recurrent parotid swellings.

Recurrent Sialadenitis (Parotid): This chronic disorder is due to the interplay between three underlying aetiological factors, namely obstruction of the duct, hyposecretion and ascending infection, which are frequently closely interwoven so that which is ultimately most important in a given case often cannot be discerned. The emphasis given to each factor has changed recently from infection (Rose, 1954) to obstruction and hyposecretion (Patey, 1965 and Maynard, 1965). It is simplest to discuss each factor separately before considering the pathology and clinical features.

Pathogenesis and pathology

(i) *Obstruction* of the parotid duct may be due to inflammatory swelling of its orifice on the parotid papilla which is seen particularly in the elderly due to irritation of a denture and this may be followed by a stricture of the duct orifice.

Calculi within the parotid duct occur not infrequently, being recognized about one-third as often as in the submandibular duct, according to Patey. Calculi may lead to stricture of the duct, as may infection and operation for the recovery of a duct stone. Rarely duct obstruction is due to a neoplasm pressing upon the duct.

Obstruction of the parotid duct leads to a very substantial reduction in the secretion of saliva and for this reason is not necessarily associated with postprandial swelling. Swelling tends to be irregular and is probably more associated with infection. It may be relieved by massage of the gland which causes a gush of saliva and debris.

(ii) *Hyposecretion:* This, as noted above, may follow duct obstruction due to various causes. A purely endogenous cause is the destruction of acinar tissue which occurs in the sicca syndrome. This may be associated with parotid swelling due to the underlying disease, but not uncommonly forms the basis for recurrent ascending infection which is the cause of the patient's symptoms.

This syndrome is associated with the characteristic sialographic finding of punctate sialectasis and, as will be described later, is almost certainly auto-immune in origin. Patey describes this as being associated with recurrent sialo-adenitis in 38 per cent of cases, but in Maynard's series only 10 per cent progressed to the complete syndrome. Although parotid flow is reduced bilaterally in this disease, symptoms of recurrent sialo-adenitis are almost invariably unilateral.

(iii) *Infection:* Ascending infection of the parotid duct follows duct obstruction or hyposecretion and is the proximate cause of symptoms in most cases. It is, or course, associated with further glandular destruction although the organisms involved are not of great pathogenicity, being the normal oral flora (*S. viridans, S. faecalis, S. albus*).

Infection may lead to mucous hyperplasia, duct metaplasia and be associated with stone formation.

It thus follows that there is a cycle of events which tends to be self-perpetuating in the production of this syndrome. In any case it may be difficult to decide which was the original cause of the disease.

The principal histological features include acinar destruction with fibrosis and patchy inflammatory cellular exudate. Ducts may be dilated and contain pus and the major ducts show hyperplasia of mucous glands and squamous metaplasia of the epithelial lining.

Clinical features

The symptoms are unilateral and consist initially of swelling with pain, but trismus is slight. At this stage the diagnosis is not made but becomes apparent as recurrent attacks occur. The swelling lasts for 2–10 days and attacks recur at intervals of several weeks or months.

Examination reveals a tender elastic swelling which is pre-auricular, the overlying skin being normal. The duct orifice may be inflamed and there is lack of salivary secretion while massage of the gland may cause passage of thick flocculent debris followed by a gush of saliva.

Radiography in the postero-anterior plane and of the anterior portion of the duct by means of a dental film held in the cheek reveals stones, if present.

Sialography should be performed in each case in an interval between acute attacks and may reveal main duct dilatation, stricture, radiolucent filling defect (radiolucent stone), punctate sialectasis (sicca syndrome) or, in the most advanced cases, complete disorganization. Abnormal findings may be confined to a branch duct and its tributaries.

Estimation of flow rates is advisable but still rather experimental, the flow from the diseased gland being compared with the contralateral gland. A Lashley canula is applied to each duct and saliva collected while chewing gum or after intravenous injection of pilocarpine. The normal flow is about 1·0 ml per minute and in most cases the diseased gland will show a marked reduction, although this is frequently bilateral.

In cases with an underlying sicca syndrome symmetrical reduction of secretion is to be expected.

The prognosis is related to the secretion rate; being better when secretion is normal in volume or slightly depressed.

Treatment

In all cases it is prudent to dilate the duct orifice for as far as is possible with a series of lacrimal probes.

Stones in the oral part of the duct may be removed from an incision on to the duct from the oral mucosa. The more deeply placed stones required excision via a linear external incision.

In cases with no obvious remediable cause, stimulation of secretion by means of chewing gum is called for. Acute episodes may be controlled by a combination of antibiotics and gland massage. In severe cases, symptoms may only be controlled by either duct ligation or superficial parotidectomy.

Duct ligation is only performed when marked hyposecretion is present, i.e. where the sicca syndrome is basically at fault or gland destruction is far advanced. Where secretion rate is high parotidectomy is indicated.

Recurrent Sialadenitis (Submandibular): This is a commoner clinical presentation than recurrent parotid swelling and is closely associated with obstruction of the submandibular duct by a stone. The obstruction is usually only partial and so symptoms typically consist of postprandial pain and swelling of the involved gland. Ascending infection may, on occasion, produce acute sialadenitis in an obstructed gland, but is not common.

Rarely recurrent swelling is due to a neoplasm in the gland which causes duct obstruction.

Examination usually reveals an enlarged firm submandibular salivary gland and swelling can be reproduced by asking the patient to think of his favourite meal or to suck a lemon. This also demonstrates lack of flow of saliva from the affected duct.

Radiographic examination in the lateral oblique position and the occlusal view of the floor of the mouth reveal the stone.

Treatment consists of removal of the stone if it lies above the mylohyoid muscle or removal of the gland if the stone is beyond the reach of an intra-oral approach. Excision of the gland is also necessary if recurrent severe symptoms occur. These, as is demonstrable on sialography, are associated with widespread glandular destruction and duct sialectasis which probably originated in infection or stricture of the duct.

Occasionally, acute infection occurs in the obstructed gland and treatment with antibiotics (penicillin being the drug of choice) is required before definitive treatment can be undertaken.

Sicca Syndrome: *Syn.* Sjögren's syndrome, Gougerot's syndrome, Mikulicz's disease and syndrome, benign lympho-epithelial lesion, keratoconjunctivitis sicca, buccoglossopharyngitis sicca.

The sicca syndrome was first described in 1933 by Henrik Sjögren (a Swedish ophthalmologist) as xerophthalmia and xerostomia occurring usually in middle-aged women with rheumatoid arthritis. There may or may not be symmetrical swelling of the parotid, submandibular and lacrimal glands, but swelling is rarely marked. However, when it is severe it is striking and accounts for the cases described as Mikulicz's disease, including the original case described by Mikulicz. To cases with essentially benign sialolacrimal enlargement the term Mikulicz's disease was formerly applied to distinguish them from the similar clinical presentation where the enlargement is due to 'infiltration' in various systemic disorders such as sarcoidosis, lymphatic leukaemia and lymphosarcoma and Hodgkin's disease where, of course, the prognosis is short. These malignant counterparts ran under the all-embracing title of Mikulicz's syndrome.

As has been noted above, the sicca syndrome may be implicated in the aetiology of chronic recurrent parotid sialo-adenitis.

Thus the sicca syndrome embraces several clinical presentations which may be represented as follows:

i. 'Simple' variety—xerophthalmia, xerostomia, slight glandular swelling (common).

ii. 'Tumorous' variety in which sialolacrimal enlargement is present and if severe, was termed Mikulicz's disease.

iii. 'Complicated' variety in which ascending bacterial infection leads to sialadenitis.

Pathogenesis and pathology

The association between the sicca syndrome and another auto-immune disease, particularly rheumatoid arthritis, was noted by Sjögren, but it does also occur by itself. Even then, however, it is particularly seen in women of middle age. It is associated with a hypergammaglobulinaemia and raised sedimentation rate; all pointing to an auto-immune pathogenesis. This is largely confirmed by the histopathological findings which are described as benign lympho-epithelial lesion. The acinar tissue is destroyed but is partly replaced by a proliferation of ductal epithelium and particularly myoepithelial cells.

The lost glandular tissue is replaced by a dense infiltration of lymphoid tissue and germinal follicles may be present. The close similarity between this histological appearance and that of Hashimoto's thyroiditis was pointed out by Cardell and Gurling in 1954. Very recently it has been shown by Bertram that auto-antibodies to salivary acinar tissue are present in the blood of patients with sicca syndrome. Thus, all the evidence points strongly to the pathogenesis being auto-immune; the antigen being common to the salivary, lacrimal and other mucous glands in the body, particularly in the nose, throat and vagina.

The parallels between auto-immune thyroid disease and the sicca syndrome are striking, apart from the pathological similarity noted above. In both there is a florid form with initially little derangement of secretion (Hashimoto's and Mikulicz's disease) but the bulk of cases show extensive silent glandular destruction (Sjögren's syndrome and myxoedema). The fact that external secretion occurs in the parotid allows ascending infection of the gland which does not occur in thyroid disease. Perhaps, to extend the analogy to its limits, in the rare case of unexplained sialorrhoea an antibody corresponding to long-acting thyroid stimulator, important in the aetiology of thyrotoxicosis, will be found!

Clinical features

The commonest mode of presentation is xerostomia which, on questioning, is found to be associated with xerophthalmia and possibly dryness of the nose, throat and vagina, too. The syndrome is almost confined to females over 40 years of age and the association with other auto-immune diseases is striking. This is typically rheumatoid arthritis but may be dermatomyositis, disseminated lupus, pernicious anaemia, myxoedema or Addison's disease.

The xerostomia causes great inconvenience in eating and talking and is associated with increase in dental caries, particularly of the cervical margins.

The xerophthalmia is potentially more serious as it may be associated with conjuctival erosions and later corneal abrasions and scarring; the ocular symptoms are generally more prominent and it is noteworthy that Sjögren was an ophthalmologist.

Examination of the patient usually shows slight glandular enlargement but a number of patients never have any swelling. The mouth is dry (halitosis is common) and oral hygiene poor. The mucosa of the mouth and pharynx appears glazed and red with an atrophic look and the surface may be wrinkled. The eyes are dry and instilled Rose Bengal reveals any conjunctival abrasions.

Rarely there may be presentation with bilateral parotid or complete sialolacrimal gland enlargement but the swelling is rarely great and tends to remit after a year or two. Occasionally quite marked enlargement of minor salivary glands may be seen, particularly at the hard–soft palate junction, and the swelling causes soreness when ulcerated by the patient's denture.

As mentioned previously, a number of cases of sialo-adenitis are based in occult sicca syndrome. Minor degrees, unimportant clinically, have been noted frequently in post-mortem material by Waterhouse.

Investigations

Blood may show hypergammaglobulinaemia, high ESR, auto-antibodies to thyroid, antinuclear factor and antigammaglobulin (rheumatoid factor).

Treatment is purely symptomatic: use of a mouthwash containing 1 per cent methyl cellulose is helpful as an oral lubricant.

The eyes require 'artificial tears' (guttae 1 per cent methyl cellulose) but in the earlier stages obstruction of the lacrimal ducts may be helpful.

Mikulicz's Syndrome: As noted above, this is a term applied to cases of sialolacrimal enlargement due to disseminated disease. It may be due to sarcoidosis when the prognosis is reasonable and then may be associated with uveitis (Heerfordt's syndrome, uveoparotid fever) or facial palsy. It may also be due to lymphosarcoma, leukaemia and Hodgkin's disease, in which case the prognosis is correspondingly gloomy. It is important to exclude these before making a diagnosis of sicca syndrome, which is usually possible with clinical haematological examination, but biopsy may be necessary.

Localized Mass in Salivary Glands

The majority of localized swellings within salivary glands are neoplastic but in rare instances infection which may be tuberculous, syphilitic, fungal or pyogenic—localized to one part of the gland—is indistinguishable from a neoplasm. The true state of affairs is indicated by histological examination after excision. Adenomas and adenocarcinomas derived from salivary tissue may originate in major and minor (intraoral) salivary glands and are considered in Chapter 11.

The Mucocoele

This abnormality occurs most commonly upon the lips, cheeks or in the floor of the mouth as a soft, bluish intramucosal swelling. The history is often one of recurrent swelling and collapse. Pathologically mucocoeles are either due to extravasation of mucus from or retention of mucus in a minor salivary gland. If troublesome they may be excised.

Bibliography

Banks P. (1968) Non-neoplastic parotid swelling: a review. *Oral Surg.* **25**, 732.

Bertram U. (1967) Xerostomia. *Acta Odontol. Scand., Suppl.* **49**.

Brook A. H. (1969) Recurrent parotitis in childhood. *Br. Dent. J.* **127**, 271.

Bruce-Pearson R. S. (1961) Recurrent parotid enlargement. *Gut* **2**, 210.

Cardell B. G. and Gurling K. J. (1954) The pathology of Sjögren's syndrome. *J. Pathol. Bact.* **68**, 137.

Harrison J. D. (1975) Salivary mucocoeles. *Oral Surg.* **39**, 268.

Maynard J. D. (1965) Recurrent parotid enlargement. *Br. J. Surg.* **52**, 784.

Patey D. H. (1965) Inflammation of the salivary glands. *Ann. R. Coll. Surg.* **36**, 26.

Rose S. S. (1954) A clinical and radiological survey of 192 cases of recurrent swellings of salivary glands. *Ann. R. Coll. Surg.* **15**, 374.

Sjögren H. (1933) Zur Kenntnis der Keratoconjunctivitis. *Acta Ophthalmol. Scand., Suppl.* **2.**

Waterhouse J. P. (1966) Inflammation of the salivary glands. *Br. J. Oral Surg.* **3**, 161.

Chapter 13

Xerostomia and Ptyalism

Innervation of the salivary glands

The salivary glands have both a sympathetic and parasympathetic innervation. Parotid glands receive their parasympathetic nerve supply from the inferior salivary nucleus via the glossopharyngeal nerve to the tympanic plexus, and via the lesser superficial petrosal nerve to the otic ganglion. The submandibular and sublingual glands receive their parasympathetic nerve supply from the superior salivary nucleus via the facial nerve and the chorda tympani. Sympathetic supply to all the glands is from the superior cervical sympathetic ganglion, with the plexus of nerves reaching the salivary glands along the course of the arteries. Minor salivary glands probably also have sympathetic and parasympathetic innervations.

Neurohumoral transmission in salivary glands

Parasympathetic stimulation has a pronounced sialagogic effect. Acetylcholine is liberated at the parasympathetic ganglion and the neuro-effector junction (*Fig.* 1). At the ganglion acetylcholine has a nicotinic action and at the neuro-effector junction it has a muscarinic action. There are two stages in the production of acetylcholine:
1. The acetylation of co-enzyme A to give acetyl co-enzyme A.
2. The acetyl group from acetyl co-enzyme A is transferred to choline to give acetylcholine. This reaction requires the enzyme choline acetylase as a catalyst. Section of the parasympathetic nerve supply reduces the choline acetylase activity by 90 per cent in the salivary glands.

There is still argument about the role of sympathetic innervation to the salivary glands, and its sialogogic effect. Sympathectomy has been shown to increase the choline acetylase activity by 25 per cent. It would appear that salivary flow is regulated by a combination of sympathetic and parasympathetic effects, in the same way as is gastric secretion. There is yet one other function of the sympathetic nerve supply.

159

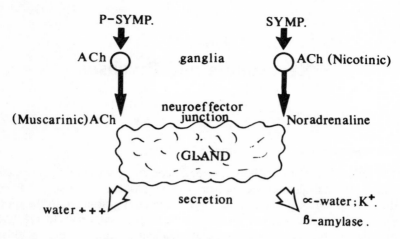

Fig. 1. Sympathetic and parasympathetic salivary neurohumoral transmission.

Acetylcholine is inactivated by the specific enzyme acetylcholinesterase and also by the non-specific enzymes cholinesterase and ben-zylcholinesterase. In some animal experiments these enzyme levels rise after sympathectomy.

Xerostomia

Xerostomia is the term used to describe an abnormally dry mouth, in the same way as xerophthalmia can be used for a dry eye and xerodermia for a dry skin. Where there is dryness of mucosa in a number of areas, such as eye, mouth, nose and pharynx, the term sicca syndrome is often used. Individual areas of mucosal dryness can be referred to as keratoconjunc-tivitis sicca, rhinitis sicca, pharyngitis sicca and even laryngitis sicca. In each of these cases it may be possible to demonstrate dryness of the mucosa, but there are many cases where the dryness is subjective.

In the mouth the mucosa normally has a moist shiny appearance. If dried with a piece of gauze beads of moisture will appear from the local glands within a few minutes. These glands, important though they may be, only produce a very small part of the total lubricant for the mouth, the majority being produced by the major salivary glands. The parotid glands are most important in this respect. It is possible for a patient to have both submandibular glands removed without much difficulty after the operation, but even the removal of one parotid gland, or the loss of its secretion, results in some dryness of the mouth.

Causes of xerostomia

1. *Physiological:* The subjective sensation of a dry mouth will follow excessive speaking and during exercise. Two factors are in operation under these circumstances. Mouth breathing which occurs in exercise, speaking or singing will have a drying effect on the mouth. There is also an emotional component which causes sympathetic stimulation of the autonomic nervous system and some suppression of the parasympathetic system, the net result being diminished salivary flow and a dry mouth. Most people have experienced the dry mouth sensation before an important interview or before rising to make an important speech.

2. *Agenesis of salivary glands:* This is extremely rare, but occasionally patients are seen who from birth have had dry mouths. Sialography may demonstrate major defects of the salivary glands. There are varying degrees of this condition. Minor symptoms consist of difficulty in eating dry food and a constant feeling of dryness of the mouth. In major cases there will be the appearance of dry mucosa, with a red, inflamed but dry looking, tongue. The dental caries rate is very much increased. Conservation of teeth is important as these patients find it is very difficult to wear dentures.

3. *Due to nasal obstruction:* In children the most common cause of nasal obstruction is enlarged nasopharyngeal tonsils (adenoids). In adults there are a variety of causes from deviated nasal septum, nasal polyps or even a hypertrophic rhinitis. All these conditions will cause the patient to breathe through his mouth. Many children develop the habit of breathing through the mouth without nasal obstruction. There may be a malocclusion of the incisors, usually protruding upper incisors (Angle's Class II, Division 1 malocclusion), or the lips are weak and incompetent. These two factors may be seen together.

No matter the cause, the result is the same: a subjective feeling of a dry mouth and hyperplasia of the dry gingival tissues arounds the upper incisors on the labial surface. This may become shiny, red and will often bleed easily.

Treatment consists of first finding the causative factor and correcting that before turning to the mouth itself. A simple test for nasal obstruction is to ask the patient to breathe through his nose. Some will not be able to do this and become distressed at the effort; this would indicate complete nasal obstruction. Others will breathe through the nose with difficulty in the same way as a patient with a common cold. A small wisp of cotton wool held by the nostrils in turn will indicate if they are patent. Allergic rhinitis will give some seasonal incidence but can persist for a long time. Antihistamines will help if a diagnosis can be made with certainty, otherwise the services of an ENT surgeon must be enlisted. As a temporary measure the gingivae should be kept moist, especially at night. A silicone jelly will help in this respect.

Night is the most common time for people to breathe through the mouth. A dry mouth in the morning does not indicate nasal obstruction in the pathological sense. A patient lying on his back may snore, which is due to the soft palate being allowed to fall back like a curtain into the way of inspired and especially expired air. This may in effect cause nasal obstruction and the resulting mouth breathing will leave the patient with a dry mouth. Salivary flow is also diminished at night and vivid dreams can increase sympathetic tone. Thus a patient, lying on his back at night, may snore, have vivid dreams and awake with a dry mouth.

4. *Ageing factors and psychological factors:* Subjectively the mouth becomes dryer with advancing age, which is borne out by the fact that many old people find that their mouth gives them perplexity in this respect. This may either show itself with difficulty in eating and swallowing, or in problems over dentures. Dry mucosa makes the wearing of dentures very uncomfortable, by failing to provide that thin layer of mucus on which the denture almost floats over the surface, and with less surface tension the retention of an upper denture becomes a torment. Once the denture-bearing surface becomes sore, the trauma becomes perpetuated.

There is another group of patients, often women in the menopausal age group, but men of this age group are not immune, who complain bitterly about various sensations in their mouths, of which dryness is only one. On examination these patients have no objective features of dryness of the mouths. Many bottles of glycerine of thymol mouth-wash have been dispensed in an attempt to appease such patients. Patients of this type with obsessional features, which among other things means that they will constantly return for more treatment, are a constant worry to both doctors and dentists. There is no real treatment known for these patients but patience and ingenuity of treatment, provided that there are no harmful side effects. Many of these patients will be quite satisfied as long as they are given a sympathetic consultation, a superficial examination and an impressive bottle of coloured mouth-wash. It is surprising that many of such patients have enough insight into their condition to know that the prescribed remedy does little for their condition, but are quite happy to continue returning for more.

Other patients of this type have more florid psychiatric features either of a mild depression or of an anxiety state. Treatment with anti-depressants or tranquillizers can be rewarding in selected cases.

5. *Xerostomia in fevers and respiratory infections:* Quite non-specifically a fever will produce a dry mouth; usually this is only a minor nuisance to the patient and can be relieved by frequent sips of water. In debilitated patients a dry mouth often becomes secondarily infected with *Candida albicans,* and there is a danger of ascending parotid infection resulting in acute suppurative parotitis.

Respiratory infections usually produce a dry mouth. In the case of upper respiratory infections blockage of the nose causes mouth breathing. Bronchitis, asthma and pneumonia cause dyspnoea with usually an increased respiratory rate, and in the patient's effort to get as much ventilation as possible he breathes through the mouth. In asthmatics particularly, the mouth becomes very dry with inspissated mucus deposited round the teeth.

Oral hygiene is very important in preventing secondary infection. This will be aided by keeping the mouth moist. Even if the pneumonia is a terminal condition one of the humanities that can be offered the patient is the relief of xerostomia.

6. *Diseases of salivary glands producing xerostomia:* Apart from Sjögren's syndrome which is described separately, diseases of the salivary glands rarely cause xerostomia. The disease would need to involve both parotid glands simultaneously for gross effects to be present. Mumps is one of the few conditions that gives transient bilateral parotid inflammation and, as would be expected, there may be a short period of xerostomia in severe cases of bilateral mumps. Parotitis of the ascending type can also cause xerostomia.

7. *Sicca syndrome (Sjögren's syndrome):* This is the most important cause of xerostomia and its features have been considered in the preceding chapter. Typically the patient is female, menopausal and suffers from another auto-immune disease, typically rheumatoid arthritis.

Many other mucosae other than the mouth may be involved. The oral mucosa has a dry wrinkled or glazed appearance and a specific 'lobulation' of the tongue may occur.

8. *Following radiotherapy:* With new and better radiotherapy, even when irradiating the mouth it is possible to protect the salivary glands and prevent damage. Irradiation of the parotid is rarely needed. Even following unilateral irradiation of a parotid gland there can be marked changes. In younger patients with natural teeth, the dental caries incidence rises rapidly. Usually this is a cervical type of caries which can involve every tooth. It is amazing to see how almost exactly half of the mouth can be affected, with the mucosa appearing dry and caries extending to the midline.

9. *Other conditions causing xerostomia:* Uncontrolled diabetes mellitus with associated polydypsia and polyuria will produce a dry mouth. Diabetes insipidus will by virtue of its dehydrating nature cause xerostomia. Any case of medical or surgical dehydration will have the same effect; this covers a wide range of conditions from haemorrhage to hyperparathyroidism. Uraemia not only gives a foul tasting mouth but will produce xerostomia. Heavy smoking may produce ptyalism initially but after a few hours there will be a dry mouth.

10. *Drug-induced xerostomia:* There is a wide range of drugs which produce as one of their side effects xerostomia. To mention all the drugs where a dry mouth has been reported would almost require reproduction of the pharmacopoeia. A few drugs from each group will be mentioned in association with which xerostomia is commonly encountered.

a. DRUGS ACTING ON HIGHER CENTRES OF THE BRAIN. All drugs which depress the activity of the higher centres of the brain will also depress the sympathetic and parasympathetic nervous system. The anti-sialagogic effect is analogous to the diminution of salivary flow in sleep. This will to some degree cover all drugs which fall into the vague categories of sedatives, hypnotics, narcotics and tranquillizers.

b. DRUGS ACTING ON AUTONOMIC GANGLIA: The action here is predominantly via the parasympathetic ganglia, which have the same neurohumoral mode of transmission as the sympathetic ganglia. Nicotine causes initial stimulation followed in high doses by blockade. Thus in theory heavy smokers should suffer from xerostomia. Certainly this is backed by clinical impression, but it is impossible to say how much of this is due to local changes in the oral mucosa.

Ganglion-blocking agents are rarely needed now in the control of hypertension. One of the reason that they have been superseded by more specific drugs was that they produced a number of side effects (one of which was xerostomia). It is occasionally necessary to use drugs like mecamylamine, pempidine and pentolinium in the control of sudden hypertension, and when these drugs are used the patients will always complain of xerostomia and blurred vision.

c. DRUGS ACTING ON THE PARASYMPATHETIC NEURO-EFFECTOR JUNC-TION: The majority of drugs which cause xerostomia act at this site by blocking the muscarinic effects of acetylcholine. Atropine, its natural alkaloid belladonna, together with related substances such as homatropine, hyoscine and their quarternary ammonium products, have the effect of drying the mouth if given systemically. A number of drugs used as spasmolytics and to reduce gastric acid secretion, such as propantheline (Probanthene) and poldine (Nacton) have a similar effect.

All antihistamines have cholinergic side effects and reduce salivary flow. Phenothiazine derivatives have the same effect; in fact many of the antihistamines are phenothiazine derivatives. The same applies to many of the drugs which are used for the treatment of Parkinsonism, such as benzhexol, benztropine and orphenadrine.

The tricyclic antidepressants such as imipramine, amitriptyline and their related compounds may produce a dry mouth. As endogeneous depression in its own right produces xerostomia, it may be difficult to decide if the disease or its treatment is producing the dry mouth.

d. DRUGS ACTING AT THE ADRENERGIC NEURO-EFFECTOR JUNCTION: Amphetamine and its numerous derivatives, which are used as stimulants or even as appetite depressants, will to a limited degree reduce salivary flow. Ephedrine, which may still be used in asthma to relieve bronchospasm, will have a similar effect. Fortunately bronchial dilators are being produced which have a more specific effect and less action on the salivary glands.

Treatment of xerostomia

Mild cases can be treated with frequent drinks, and the patient may find it advantageous to have a glass of water by the bedside or to aid the swallowing of food. Mouth-washes such as glycerine of thymol have a place in selected cases. The colour and smell even appeals to the simpler patients. A 1 per cent methyl cellulose mouth-wash will be helpful in severe cases; there is no harm in the patient swallowing the solution as it may even help the passage of food down the oesophagus.

Drugs with a specific parasympathetic stimulating effect are both dangerous and ineffective. This is not surprising where the xerostomia is due to damage of salivary tissue. Pilocarpine drops may have limited effect in some cases.

Ptyalism

For patients with bulbar palsy as part of motor neurone disease, the lack of swallowing and the incompetence of the lips leads to the miserable picture of a patient sitting, expressionless, with his head forward, dribbling down his chest. It is doubtful if there is any real increase in salivary flow.

Parkinsonian patients may also suffer from uncontrolled salivation. Again, this may be accentuated by the facial immobility. Most of the anti-Parkinsonian drugs have an anti-sialogic effect.

'Water-brash' is a sudden flow of saliva into the mouth. Often there is no cause for this, but occasionally it is associated with disease of the upper part of the alimentary tract. Patients with an oesophageal stricture will in severe cases have difficulty in swallowing their saliva.

Patients wearing partial dentures for the first time often find there is an increased flow of saliva. Any foreign body in the mouth has a sialogic effect. Full denture wearers do not seem to suffer from this disability. A lesion of the oral mucosa, especially if it is voluminous like a fungating carcinoma, will caused increased production of saliva. Carcinoma of the tongue is notorious for this, but even severe periodontal diseases can have sialogic effects.

Mercurial and iodide preparations are drugs which have little use in modern therapy but produce increased salivary flow. Drugs are used to make sputum loose, such as various so-called expectorant mixtures. Ipecacuanha, ammonium chloride, ammonium bicarbonate and squill will all have the same effect and are still used by some medical practitioners; in addition to increasing sputum they do increase salivary flow.

Occasionally patients are encountered who become obsessional about their salivary flow, claiming that they are constantly having to swallow their saliva, a function that most of us achieve hundreds of times a day without noticing it. Some patients with periodontal disease will even present with a sample of bloodstained saliva in a little bottle. Such patients need reassurance and correction of their minor pathology, but by the nature of their personality these patients are often very persistent.

Treatment of ptyalism

In such cases as motor neurone disease ptyalism can be a very distressing feature of their disease. Belladonna drops may help to some degree, and at least this is one aspect of this very distressing disease for which some rational symptomatic treatment can be given. In other cases of ptyalism it is a matter of finding the aetiological factor and if possible removing it.

Some patients salivate excessively when they attend the dentist. Atropine or belladonna could be used in small doses, but one of the simplest treatments is to give propantheline 15 mg an hour before treatment. Two of the side effects of antihistamines could be used to produce a dry mouth and to sedate the patient. Promethazine hydrochloride in a dose of 50 mg would be needed or a high dose of one of the other antihistamines.

Bibliography

Burgen A. S. V. and Emmelin N. G. (1961) *The Physiology of Salivary Glands,* London, Arnold.

Ellman P. et al. (1951) A contribution to the pathology of Sjögren's syndrome. *Q. J. Med.* **20,** 33.

Goodman L. S. and Gillman A. (1965) *The Pharmacological Basis of Therapeutics,* 3rd ed. New York, Macmillan.

Schneyer L. H. and Schneyer C. A. (1967) *Secretory Mechanisms of Salivary Glands,* New York, Academic Press.

Todd R. G. (1967) *Extra Pharmacopoeia,* 25th ed. London, Pharmaceutical Press.

Chapter 14

Halitosis and Cacogeusia

There are a number of confusing terms related to offensive odours of the breath and disagreeable tastes in the mouth. It is best to start by defining the various terms in use.

Cacogeusia—from the Greek *kakos* (bad) and *geusis* (taste). This generally refers to a bad taste in the mouth which has arisen independent of diet.

Halitosis—from the Latin *halitus* (breath) and the Greek *osis* (condition). Thus, literally, halitosis is a condition of the breath. Generally this is taken to mean offensive breath.

Foetor (meaning foul odour) may be used relating to the breath in the following ways:

foetor ex ore—an odour from the mouth

foetor oris—an odour of the mouth

foetor narium—an odour from the nose

foetor hepaticum—an odour of the breath which is said to be specific for liver disease.

Ozaena—an unpleasant odour specifically from the nose, generally related to nasal pathology.

Hyperosmia—an increased sensitiveness to odour. This can occur in psychiatric states, but on rare occasions may be associated with a lesion causing irritation of the olfactory apparatus.

Cacosmia—this is where the patient has the perception of an evil odour in his own nose, but it can also be a subjective sensation or even the aura of epilepsy.

Parosmia—this is the perception of imagined odours and is always of central origin, usually associated with psychiatric states, but it may be part of the aura of epilepsy.

Of these terms, probably the most accurate for an odour of the breath is foetor ex ore, but halitosis is the traditional term used. Some cases of halitosis may be associated with cacogeusia, while elsewhere the two conditions occur independently.

Measurements of Odour

There is marked observer error in assessment of odour of the breath. There have been attempts to make this more scientific, but all methods depend on personal observation. From the experimental point of view it is possible to measure odour by means of a cryoscope and osmoscope. The subject breathes into a tube connected to a condenser surrounded by liquid nitrogen (a *cryoscope*) and the breath is frozen. At a later stage the condenser containing the frozen breath is placed in a water bath at body temperature. From the heated condenser a tube runs to the observer's nostrils. There is a side limb which acts as an air inlet. This second apparatus is an *osmoscope*. By adjusting the air inlet dilutions can be made, so that the odour is only just detectable. This may be expressed as a minus logarithm of the dilution and is called the pO. Readings have been recorded with human breath ranging from pO 0–6 with an average pO of 2. Some workers have dispensed with the cryoscope and made direct measurements with the osmoscope.

It must be stressed that these measurements are not in routine use but are solely of experimental value and depend on the same observer being used in each case.

Causes of Odours arising from the Mouth

Most cases of halitosis or cacogeusia fall into this group. Many of the causes are so common that they must be regarded as the norm.

'Morning breath'

There is generally an odour from the breath and a taste first thing in the morning. This is due to the lack of salivation during the night and the failure of movements of the mouth to remove desquamated epithelium. There may be some putrefaction of the debris during the night. Saliva very soon putrefies, as can easily be demonstrated. Excessive mouth breathing or snoring during the night will make this worse. After a meal or after cleaning the teeth the 'morning breath' disappears. Halitosis from any other cause will be at its worst first thing in the morning.

'Hunger breath'

Hunger can cause halitosis and claims have been made that this is due to hypoglycaemia; this, while not proven, is certainly cured by a meal.

Diet

The diet itself can be a factor in halitosis; fried food will give an odour even after the teeth have been cleaned and tea and coffee also have a characteristic odour and taste, but this usually disappears following the use of a toothbrush. Many highly-spiced foods cause foetor ex ore, but a number of these odours are due to excretion of volatile substances from the lungs and will be discussed later.

'Smoker's breath'

The odour and taste from smoking are characteristic and it is generally possible to tell whether the patient has been smoking cigarettes, cigars or a pipe. Patients who inhale will exude the odour from lungs, bronchi, mouth, nose and paranasal sinuses; increased mucus secretion makes this worse.

Pathological conditions of the mouth causing foetor oris

Poor oral hygiene: This is the most obvious cause of foetor oris and cacogeusia and tends to be worse in smokers with nicotine-stained deposits of calculus on the teeth. Some patients have a tendency to form calculus quickly and this may be associated with foetor oris.

Periodontal conditions: These are perhaps the most common pathologies to give rise to foetor oris and cacogeusia. It may be for this reason alone that the breath of a young child or even a young animal has a sweet odour or no odour at all, but as age advances with the human being and even to some degree in animals the odour of the breath tends to become unpleasant as periodontal disease advances and debris collects between the teeth. Frank pus formation in pyorrhoea gives cacogeusia and even foetor ex ore.

Degenerating blood in the mouth: Whatever its cause, be it from bleeding gums, post-tonsillectomy or post-oral surgery, produces a salty taste and a characteristic odour.

Vincent's infection: This will give rise to an odour which is said to resemble rotten hay. Suffice it to say that it has a characteristically repulsive odour and taste.

Gross caries: This can on occasions be detected and is generally part of the odour of a neglected mouth.

Dentures: These, too, can have an offensive odour if they are not kept scrupulously clean. Vulcanite dentures are now always old and generally rather offensive, but even acrylic dentures can develop an odour which is not pleasant.

Ulcer and tumours: Virtually any oral lesion will give rise to foetor. Pericoronitis, ulcers and malignant tumours are all associated with foetor.

Furred tongue: Even in a child, a furred tongue is offensive. A black hairy tongue often causes the patient to complain of cacogeusia.

Conditions of the nasopharynx

Septic conditions of the nose and associated structures usually give rise to ozaena, but a postnasal drip from sinusitis will give rise to cacogeusia. Rhinitis is rarely the cause of ozaena, but sinusitis is the most frequent cause. Septic adenoids and tonsils can give rise to nasal obstruction with foetor ex ore or cacogeusia. Even pharyngitis can give halitosis and cacogeusia. Cacogeusia is a common sequel to respiratory infections and influenza. Post-tonsillectomy there will be the same odour of decaying blood which is to be expected after oral surgery.

Conditions arising from the lungs and bronchi

Diseases of the lungs and bronchi where abscesses, cavities and areas of stagnation occur will give rise to a very offensive odour from the breath. Such conditions as bronchiectasis, lung abscesses, empyema and any condition which causes lung cavitation give a stench to the breath which on occasions can pervade the room the patient is in.

Conditions of the alimentary tract

It used to be considered that conditions of the upper part of the alimentary tract, such as peptic ulceration, caused halitosis. As the oesophagus is normally a collapsed tube and is shut off from the stomach by a competent gastro-oesophagal sphincter, no odour from the stomach can escape except during flatulence. Even in cases with severe pyloric stenosis the rule does not seem to be broken. Gross pathology of the stomach such as a carcinoma will manifest only intermittently until its terminal stages, when there is probably another reason for the halitosis. It is remarkable how little odour there is from a condition of the oesophagus. Even achalasia of the cardia rarely produces foetor ex ore and the same would apply to oesophageal spasm (corkscrew oesophagus). A pharyngeal pouch is not noted for its foetor.

It has been claimed that there is a characteristic foetor from the breath of a patient who is bleeding from the alimentary tract. Generally there is an aroma of malaena surrounding the bed of the patient, but this is more often from flatus coupled with lack of oral hygiene and solid food. Constipation used to be cited as a common cause of halitosis, but this has been disproved in volunteers who were made constipated by drugs.

Dehydration

All conditions which cause dehydration will also cause foetor ex ore. Even drying of the mouth will have this effect in such physiological states as sleep, mouth breathing and heavy exercise or prolonged public speaking. After a general anaesthetic the halitosis is quite marked, due to the inactivity and to the action of atropine. This can be well illustrated by doing a postoperative ward round on patients who have had operations excluding the mouth.

Foetor hepaticum

This is certainly present in severe acute liver failure and may be taken as a sign that coma is about to supervene, if it has not already done so. Foetor hepaticum has been described by a number of terms as being 'amine-like', 'musty', 'mousey', and claims have been made that the aroma is that of a fresh corpse. Neurological features of liver failure and foetor hepaticum tend to occur together and may even have a common aetiology. Both tend to remit as the condition responds to treatment. Although it has been claimed that foetor hepaticum may be present in conditions other than acute liver failure, e.g. cirrhosis and cholecystitis, this has not been substantiated; the odour may be due to other causes existing simultaneously.

Foetor oris in chronic renal failure

The mouth generally becomes foul in advanced renal failure, with a dry, discoloured tongue and even a stomatitis. Urea is excreted via the salivary glands when the patient is severely uraemic and the breath may have a urine-like smell.

Substances excreted via the lungs

A number of volatile substances are excreted via the expired air from the lungs. These substances are present in the bloodstream and pass across the capillary alveolar membrane.

Ketones: In a diabetic crisis there are high concentrations of ketones in the blood, giving ketosis. Acetoacetic acid, hydroxybutyric acid and acetone are all present. Acetone has a sweet, aromatic odour which may be detected at the bedside of the patient by the clinician with a good sense of smell.

Paraldehyde: This can be detected in the same way and will even pervade the ward. Before the use of more modern drugs, this smell was dominant in psychiatric wards.

Disulfiram (Antabuse): This is used as a deterrent to alcoholics by converting alcohol to aldehyde and will give halitosis and cacogeusia in alcoholics even if they are not taking alcohol.

Food substances absorbed from the alimentary tract and excreted from the mouth

There are a number of food substances which give rise to halitosis which not only leave an odour and a taste in the mouth, but are also excreted through the lungs. Garlic, alcohol, onions, radishes and the like fall into this group. Various experiments have been performed to prove this with garlic. It is possible to give a subject a capsule containing garlic and by so doing the garlic reaches the stomach or duodenum before it is released. Even in these cases the odour of garlic can be detected as a foetor ex ore. It has also been claimed that it is possible to rub garlic into the soles of the feet with the same result. The whole basis of breath tests by the police relates to the fact that alcohol is excreted in the breath.

Menstruation

Various odours have been described from the breath premenstrually and during the menstrual period described as 'mousey' or even that of decaying blood. Attempts have been made to correlate this with attraction of the opposite sex in more primitive animals. The converse is more likely to be true in man, but there is no parallel between man and the rest of the animal kingdom due to variation in ovulation in relation to menstruation. Animals may emit an odour which may be detected a mile away by the opposite sex of the same species, but this is not necessarily from the mouth.

Neuroses related to halitosis and cacogeusia

There is no doubt that noticeable halitosis is a great social stigma and can lead to social ostracism. This in itself is enough to make a patient at least very sensitive over the question of halitosis. A number of patients present with a variety of complaints where the basic underlying problem is loss of libido by their sexual partner which may be due to the patient's own halitosis or alleged halitosis. This aspect of the case should never be overlooked in cases where no detectable halitosis is noted on a number of occasions. Also, the possibility of halitosis being a paranoid delusion must be entertained. The patient thinks that while talking to him other people turn their heads away or put their hand to their face to protect themselves from the odour. This is true for halitosis, cacogeusia and cacosmia. It is very difficult, if not impossible, to prove that a patient's cacogeusia is functional. Much time and effort can be spent in investigation with negative results; it is only when other bizarre complaints are made by the patient that a functional diagnosis seems certain. Olfactory delusions are not usually seen in psychotic states, but may be the aura of epilepsy.

Investigation and diagnosis: In outpatient practice renal, hepatic or diabetic causes are not likely to be seen. The most common are oral, nasal and psychological causes. Psychological causes can be excluded by detection of the odour. It may be useful to check this discreetly with a colleague, as one observer may have a poor sense of smell, especially for this particular odour. Oral causes are the most common, but should these be absent, then nasal causes should be sought and, lastly, causes from the lungs. It may be possible to detect the odour solely from the nose or solely from the mouth. A careful history helps considerably and may remove the necessity for prolonged investigation.

Causes such as diet, 'smoker's breath', 'morning breath' and menstrual breath must be specifically considered if they are to be diagnosed.

Treatment

Basically the treatment of halitosis or cacogeusia is the treatment of the underlying condition. Particular attention should be paid to oral hygiene, especially after meals. Various toothpastes and other preparations may be used to cover up the odour, but this should not be regarded as treatment. In some cases, even after prolonged investigation no cause can be found and these measures form the last resort. The most difficult cases to treat are those in which a psychological factor is present and the patient has become obsessional and even hypersensitive about his breath. Professional reassurance may help in a limited number of cases. A frank discussion with the patient about the problem is usually the best approach. Point out to the patient the factors which can cause halitosis in normal everyday life, such as 'morning breath', diet with special reference to foetor ex ore after a meal or a beverage and explain that cleaning the teeth at this time will be all that is needed.

Bibliography

Hine M. K. (1957) Halitosis. *JAMA* **55**, 37.

Massler M., Emslie R. D. and Bolden T. G. (1951) Fetor-ex-ore. *Oral Surg.* **4**, 110.

Morris P. P. and Read R. R. (1949) Halitosis. *J. Dent. Res.* **28**, 324.

McNamara T. F. Alexander J. F. and Lee M. (1972) The role of microorganisms in the production of oral malodor. *Oral Surg.* **34**, 41.

Spouge J. D. (1964) Halitosis, a review of its cause and treatment. *Dent. Pract.* **14**, 307.

Chapter 15

Facial Pain. I

Introduction

Pain, although the most common symptom in many branches of medicine and virtually the *raison d'être* of dental surgery, is very poorly understood at the physiological level. Pain may be thought of in a strictly neurological sense and, certainly when considering the control of pain provoked by operative procedures, this approach has value. In many instances, however, where pain is associated with psychological disorders, it is said to be impossible to explain it on the basis of evoked peripheral changes secondarily perceived as pain, although this mechanism is implied or even explicitly described. Thus pain perceived as headache may be described as resulting from tension or stress which causes 'muscle spasm' with or without vascular changes which themselves are the ultimate cause of pain. Where even this psychosomatic concept falls down we may complain to the patient that the pain is imaginary or in the mind.

It is true, however, that no pain exists outside the experience of the patient, and there is no observable correlate by means of which we can check that pain is or is not being felt. Thus in dealing with pain we are in much the same situation as, for instance, the clinician faced with 'anaemia' (as a clinical observation) in the absence of any haematological tests.

In this state of woeful ignorance we must accept at face value the patient's statement that he is in pain; thus the pain associated with acute inflammation of the dental pulp is no more (or less) real than pain of 'psychological' origin (Merskey and Spear, 1967).

The face, underlying oral and nasal cavities, and the associated structures are supplied with sensory nerve fibres by the trigeminal nerve. The posterior third of the tongue and faucial region are supplied by the glossopharyngeal nerve and the skin corresponding to these regions over the angle of the mandible is supplied by the upper cervical nerves. The peripheral distribution of nerve fibres in the face will not be considered but a résumé of the central pain pathways is appended (Wyke, 1968).

Anatomy (*Fig.* 2)

The cell bodies of the first order neurones form the trigeminal ganglion, their axons forming the peripheral branches of the nerve and their central processes the sensory root which enters the pons. Within the brain stem the pain fibres become dissociated from those of common sensation and descend to synapse with the cells of the spinal nucleus.

The fibres derived from the ophthalmic division synapse with the most inferior cells of the spinal nucleus (adjacent to the dorsal horn cells of the first cervical nerve) while those of the mandibular division synapse at its upper end with the fibres of the maxillary division between.

The fibres of the spinal nucleus cells travel upward in the contralateral bulbothalamic tract (a few are ipsilateral) to the ventrolateral nucleus of the thalamus. Third order neurones transmit onward from the thalamus to the hypothalamus and one of three cerebral cortical areas: the postcentral gyrus of the parietal lobe, the orbital surface of the frontal lobe and the temporal lobe.

It is likely that each of these three sites is associated with analysis of different facets of the painful experience. The parietal cortex may be involved in analysis of the site and distribution of the stimulus, the temporal cortex with memory and the frontal cortex with the psychic reaction, the 'quality' and 'severity' of the pain. The *hypothalamic* supply explains the frequent autonomic nervous reaction to pain. Efferents from these sites also descend to the brain stem and influence the reticular-activating system whose cells are also supplied by collaterals from the sensory trigeminal afferent fibres. It is probable that the small diameter (C) pain fibres synapse not with the trigeminal nucleus but with the reticular system.

Although common sense dictates that pain is associated with certain disorders of which there is other visible or gangible evidence, the pain 'felt' may vary considerably from patient to patient and in one patient from time to time. The sites at which variations in 'sensibility' occur may be varied but the most obvious are peripheral, spinal (or brain stem) or cerebral.

At the peripheral level the proximate cause of pain, namely the actual chemical or physical stimulus which causes impulses to be transmitted along pain fibres are generally associated with cellular damage. Cellular damage, whether mediated by direct, physical, chemical, ischaemic or immunological injury, is associated with increases in local concentrations of histamine, 5-hydroxytryptamine, kinins (for example kallidin and bradykinin), prostaglandins and potassium, all of which may be

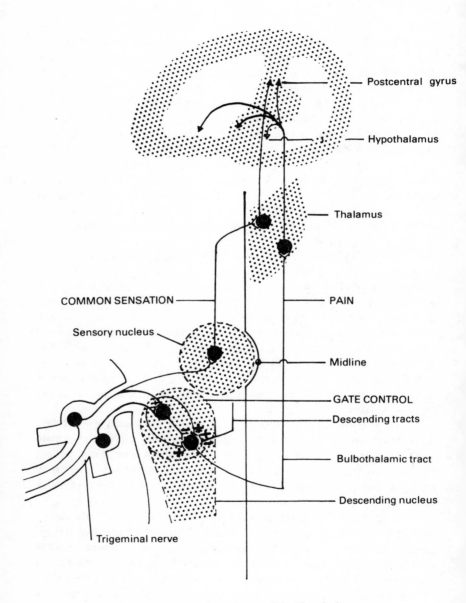

Fig. 2. Central pain pathways of the trigeminal nerve.

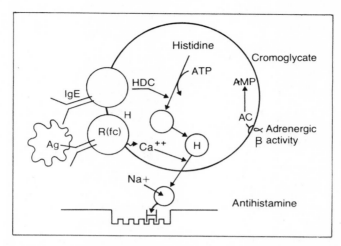

Fig. 3. The production and release of histamine. Histamine is produced from histidine by histidine decarboxylase (HDC) and stored in granules (H). The mast-cell receptor R (fc) binds IgE molecules via fc terminals leaving the antigen binding sites free. On antigen binding a change in the receptor causes intracellular calcium release (Ca^{++}) which causes the granules to be extruded. Having left the cell, the exposure of the granules to sodium in the extracellular fluid causes their rupture and so release of histamine.

associated with pain. Equally these biochemical changes are intimately associated with inflammation and blood-clotting. *Table* 1 (p. 182) illustrates some of the important interrelationships in the generation of these chemicals.

Figs. 3–5 illustrate in more detail the generation of histamine, kinins and prostaglandins. These chemicals have the ability to depolarize non-myelinated axons and thus initiate the action potential therein.

There is no doubt that considerable control over centripetal pain impulses is exercised by transactions at the level of the trigeminal nucleus in a way analogous to the gate-control as postulated by Melzak and Wall (1965). According to this the input of the A fibres synapses with trigeminal nucleus cells while collaterals pass to the adjacent reticular-activating system and thence both systems transmit onward to the cerebral cortex. The reticular formation activated by these fibres, however, inhibits the adjacent nuclear cells and thus cuts off centripetal transmission. Conversely, the C (slow) pain fibres transmit only to the reticular activating system and these are purely inhibitory and so *decrease* the inhibition exerted by these cells over nucleus cells and 'open the gate' to centripetal impulses. The reticular-activating system may also

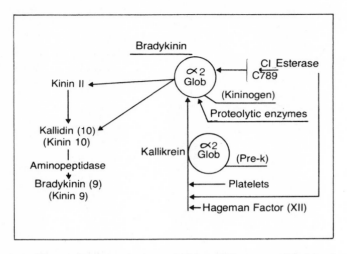

Fig. 4. The production and release of kinins. Kinins are produced by the action of proteolytic enzymes on an α_2-globulin (bradykinin). The proteolytic enzyme may be either C1 esterase or $\overline{C789}$ complex, both derived from the activation of complement, or kallikrein which is also a plasma globulin. Kallikrein is present in inactive form but may be activated by aggregated platelets or activated Hageman factor (X111a). Surface contact after extravascular spillage activates both these mechanisms. In vitro or in exceptional clinical circumstances bradykinin may be released by other proteases, i.e. snake venoms or trypsin.

be influenced by corticofugal fibres which may increase or decrease the inhibition exerted over centripetal impulses.

Although probably mediated at spinal cord or brain stem level, there is considerable control exerted by higher functions of the brain over the sensibility to pain which may be grouped together under the term 'pain threshold'. In the grip of emotion such as anger, fear or intense excitement, or in ecstatic states or hypnotic trances, stimuli normally extremely painful may pass unnoticed. At a more everyday level the preoccupation and alternative sensory input of the individual at the time of stimulus may influence the pain 'felt'.

In addition to the perception of pain there is a wide spectrum of psychic reactions to it but the reaction in any individual tends to be relatively constant and is in general accord with his psychic make-up. Thus, a phlegmatic patient may say that he feels pain but it is not of any great consequence while the nervous may find a similar stimulus excruciating and insufferable and act accordingly. The gradation from this to atypical facial pain and hysteria is but a step.

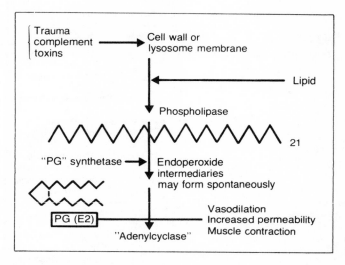

Fig. 5. The production and release of prostaglandins. Long-chain fatty acid molecules derived from cell membrane or lysosome membrane by the action of phospholipases are converted by a group of enzymes known collectively as 'prostaglandin synthetase'. It is possible that many of the steps occur spontaneously. The cell must be previously damaged for prostaglandins to appear.

In assessing facial pain a full history of site, radiation, quality, timing, precipitating or alleviating factors and associated symptoms, coupled with a full examination, serves to establish the diagnosis in the majority of cases. It must, however, constantly be borne in mind that there may be considerable similarity between pains of quite different aetiology and in difficult cases great care is necessary to establish the correct diagnosis.

It is most important to have some classification of facial pain, so that a history and examination can be carried out in a thorough fashion. One such, which is useful clinically, is to subdivide the causes basically into three groups.

1. *Pain due to local disease*

    a. Teeth and jaws.
    b. Temporomandibular joint and associated muscles.
    c. Nose and paranasal sinuses.
    d. Salivary glands.
    e. Blood vessels; giant-cell arteritis.
    f. Mucosa.
    g. Lymph nodes.

Table 1. Generation of chemicals associated with cellular damage

Antagonist	Agonist	Origin
Antihistamine	Histamine ←	Mast cell (immunological)
		Other cells (damaged)
		↑
		Peptidases (lysosymes)
		↓
—	Kinins ←	Plasma
		Globulin–kallikrein
		↑
		Activation by extravascular contact with collagen and 'foreign surfaces'
Antihistamine Methysergide	5-HT ←	'Chromaffin cells'
		Platelets
		↑
		(Aggregation on damaged vessel wall or by extravascular spillage)
Aspirin+ analogues	Prostaglandins ←	All cells
		Cell walls
		Lysosome membranes
		K+ Cell damage

In this group, the pain is associated with other symptoms and has well-defined characteristics which, with a local recognizable abnormality demonstrable clinically or radiographically, permits diagnosis. Treatment of the local condition arrests pain.

2. *Pain arising from nerve trunks and central pathways*

This group is divisible into two sub-groups, which are distinguished by the presence or absence of abnormal physical signs in the central nervous system. Thus, if the pain appears to be due to a condition belonging to this group, a prerequisite to diagnosis is a full neurological examination with particular attention directed to the cranial nerves. The causes in this group are:

Group I. No abnormal physical signs in the central nervous system.

a. Idiopathic trigeminal and glossopharyngeal neuralgia.

b. Migrainous syndromes.

c. Atypical facial pain.

Group II. Abnormal physical signs in the central nervous system.

Nerve involvement by pressure, infiltration or degenerative disease of the central nervous system, either extra- or intracranial.

3. *Pain referred from outside the face*

The pain may arise in (*a*) eyes; (*b*) ears; (*c*) heart; (*d*) cervical spine; (*e*) oesophagus.

The eyes naturally form part of the face, but normally patients do not complain of pain in the face from eye or ear disease, but complain of pain in the affected organ. Conversely, pain from other structures is commonly referred to the ear (typically from the lower molars and temporomandibular joint).

Such cases are characterized by lack of local abnormality to account for the pain, but evidence, usually fairly obvious, of disease outside the face which accounts for the pain, is found.

In the rest of this chapter will be considered pain arising in the teeth, jaws, nose and paranasal sinuses, giant-cell arteritis and pain referred from outside the face. All other subjects are covered in individual chapters.

Pain Due to Local Disease

Pain originating in the teeth and jaws

This may be subdivided as follows, according to the type of pain:
1. Hypersensitivity of the teeth (sensitive dentine).
2. Pulpitic pain.
3. Acute inflammatory pain.
4. Dull aching pain.

Hypersensitivity: The characteristics of this pain are that it is *sharp*, may be severe but lasts only a few minutes, and is always precipitated by hot, cold or sweet contact by the tooth. It is thus usually due to the presence of exposed dentine and is well localized. Exposed dentine may be discovered as a carious cavity or inadequate, cracked or leaking filling; at the neck of a tooth where gingival recession is associated with absence or acquired loss of the protective cementum; or following traumatic loss of enamel. Hypersensitivity to hot and cold (but not sweet solutions) may follow insertion of a metal filling but usually passes off in one to two weeks.

Occasionally in the reversible stage of pulpitis (particularly following the placement of a restoration in a tooth), the same symptoms may occur without exposed dentine. In this instance spontaneous pain is not a feature and the induced pain does not last more than a few minutes, which indicates that the pulp is not irreversibly affected and so remission may occur. Alternatively, pulpitis may be the sequel. If the cause cannot be found, X-rays are indicated to exclude proximal caries.

Exposed areas of dentine can be readily detected by a probe and the pain may be reproduced by application of hot or cold in the shape of either warmed gutta-percha or ethylchloride on a cotton-wool plug.

Treatment is directed to the cause. Cavities should be filled. Sometimes extraction of the offending tooth may be necessary, and defective fillings are replaced. Exposed dentine on the neck of the tooth is painted with phenol and glycerine or zinc chloride, and use of 'Sensodyne' or 'Emoform' toothpaste is a useful adjunct.

Hyperaemia of the pulp may be treated expectantly if it follows conservation, but if it does not improve in a few days a sedative dressing should be placed for a fortnight.

Pulpitic pain: This is severe pain which the patient usually recognizes as originating in a tooth, i.e. toothache, but which often cannot be localized to a particular tooth. The pain radiates into the adjacent jaw and in some cases into the ipsilateral opposite jaw.

Severe throbbing pain with paroxysmal radiation precipitated by hot or cold stimuli, but lasting for longer than ten minutes after the stimulus, is typical. Not infrequently, however, the pain may be considerably relieved by cold fluid held over the offending tooth. Spontaneous attacks of pain which may last an hour or two and be exacerbated by lying down are typical and between these severe bouts of pain, dull ache is usual which may be in the tooth or affect the whole jaw or one side of the face or may lie at some distance from the tooth, i.e. in the zygomatic region, the temporal region or the ear.

Such pulpitic pain may persist for several days, when it usually stops quite suddenly, implying necrosis of the pulp, and may then be replaced by the pain of acute inflammation due to periapical abscess.

Alternatively, such an episode lasting for a day or less may occur intermittently over quite a long period. Rarely acute pulpitic pain may be referred away completely from the tooth of origin which is asymptomatic but which is demonstrably the cause of the pain (*vide infra*).

Acute pulpitic pain is usually, as its name implies, due to acute irreversible pulpitis in a tooth. It may, however, be due to acute maxillary sinusitis where the roots of the upper posterior teeth project into the maxillary sinus. The symptoms may be almost exclusively dental and diagnostic difficulties then arise.

The dental abnormalities associated with acute pulpitic pain are usually the result of caries or its treatment and include simple caries. The tooth responsible is usually obvious, with a large cavity; but in children extensive dentinal caries may be associated with a minimal enamel lesion. Other traps are the enormous but deeply placed proximal cavities often found in upper molars, which appear to lie almost completely below gum level in relationship to deep periodontal pockets.

A peculiar form of caries has occasionally been noted in which examination of the crown reveals no abnormality, but X-ray reveals a cavity much deeper than it is wide (the reverse of usual) and originating from the neck of the tooth at the amelocemental junction. Occasionally a tooth which is the seat of acute pulpitis is noted without caries or filling, but deep periodontal pocketing is the rule. In this case, infection may travel either to the apex and infect the pulp in a retrograde fashion, or more likely the gingival recession exposes a lateral root canal which provides a route of entry for infection to the pulp.

Acute pulpitis may follow conservative treatment, either immediately or after an interval of even several years. Its development is principally related to the proximity of the pulp to the finished cavity and the trauma and heat produced by drilling and the irritating properties of filling materials. Deep silicate fillings in anterior teeth are a frequent cause of very severe pulpits. A careful history of recent fillings and their relationship to the pain is invaluable but if, as is not infrequent, the pain is diffuse and many teeth are heavily filled, great difficulty may be experienced in establishing which tooth is the seat of pain.

In such cases each tooth should be tested with hot and cold and this usually finds the culprit. Electrical pulp testing, especially in these circumstances, is very unreliable. The teeth should be tapped, for a pulpitic tooth is usually slightly periostitic.

X-rays may be taken to indicate if any teeth show unsuspected caries beneath fillings. Finally, use of diagnostic injections of local analgesics may be very helpful in localizing the tooth. In very difficult cases it may be necessary to remove all the restorations in one or two quadrants before the cause is found. Very rarely this will reveal a 'partial' fracture of a tooth which extends into the pulp chamber, a notoriously difficult source of pain to diagnose.

The treatment, of course, is to remove the pulp of the tooth, which is most readily performed by removing the whole tooth, but in suitable cases the pulp may be removed and the non-vital tooth prepared for root filling.

Pulpitic pain may, on occasion, prove difficult to distinguish from idiopathic or symptomatic neuralgia and atypical facial pain, and com-

Table 2. Main features of the four types of pain arising in teeth and jaws

	Dentine sensitivity	'Pulpitis'	Inflammatory	Nonspecific
Site	Specific tooth	Diffuse: one jaw or half-face		Diffuse
Radiation	Local	Widespread	Moderate	Local
Referral	Never	Common	Exceptional	None
Quality	Sharp	Severe (throbbing). If intermittent, dull ache persists	Persistent throbbing	Dull ache
Precipitating factors	Hot, cold, sweet	Hot (cold, sweet)	Pressure	
Relieving factors		Biting may relieve pain Pressure Cold (hot) Analgesics	Hot Analgesics	
Timing	2 minutes	Continuous or intermittent, 2–4 hours	Continuous	As pulpitic
Relation to dental treatment	+	+	+	+
Associated symptoms	−	−	Swelling	−
On examination	Exposed dentine	Caries Trauma Conservative work	Lymphadenopathy Inflammation Periostitic tooth	

plete examination as detailed above may be necessary before a local cause can be excluded.

Acute inflammatory pain: This pain is progressive, usually developing fully over 24 hours or so, and is dull, persistent, throbbing, well localized but with considerable radiation and associated with swelling and tenderness. The swelling is typically diffuse, brawny, tender and hot, and affected skin or mucosa is reddened. When it involves the muscles of mastication trismus is added to give the classical tetrad of rubor, dolor, calor and loss of function. Such acute inflammatory processes may be due to:

a. Acute periapical abscess, dental abscess, dento-alveolar abscess.
b. Acute periodontal abscess.
c. Acute pericoronitis.
d. Acute post-extraction osteitis (dry socket).
e. Acute osteomyelitis.
f. Infected dental cyst.
g. Acute sinusitis.
h. Acute cervical lymphadenitis.
i. Acute soft-tissue infections.

a. ACUTE PERIAPICAL ABSCESS: This may follow acute pulpitis but usually develops, apparently spontaneously, in connection with a tooth of which the pulp has asymptomatically necrosed, following either caries, trauma or conservative treatment. When the acute inflammatory process is contained in the jaw the pain is very severe, but rapidly extends to form an inflammatory swelling in the adjacent soft tissues and pain tends to remit somewhat. The tooth loosens and is always exquisitely tender to touch, so chewing on it is avoided. Such a tooth is said to be periostitic. In the early stages, slight reddening and tenderness of the oral mucosa over the apex of the tooth may be the only other signs. Frequently, however, very acute periapical abscess may be associated with intra-alveolar pus and the adjacent soft tissues show considerable inflammation and oedema, which if from upper incisors, may close the eye. It is not, as often termed, a cellulitis. Suppuration is early and if pus extends outside the bone it forms an abscess cavity which points within, or rarely outside, the mouth: the so-called dento-alveolar abscess. Apart from swelling, there may be trismus if a posterior tooth is the culprit. X-rays reveal an area of periapical radiolucency in most cases.

The treatment consists of drainage, which may be achieved via the root canal of the tooth or by extraction, and additional drainage of a soft tissue abscess may be necessary. Antibiotics may be given depending on the circumstances, and are useful in those situations in which immediate surgery is not possible.

b. ACUTE PERIODONTAL ABSCESS: This arises in the depths of a periodontal pocket and presents as an acute painful swelling, often on the palatal side of upper molars or in the lower incisor region. Swelling is more localized and confined to the alveolus. External swelling is very rare.

Pus can always be released by slipping college tweezers down the periodontal pocket to the abscess. The affected tooth is always loose and X-rays show irregular bone destruction due to periodontal disease.

Treatment consists either of removal of the tooth or drainage by vertical incision in the gum margin, followed by periodontal treatment, which in such cases usually involves a 'flap operation'.

c. ACUTE PERICORONITIS: As a disorder comprising more than *superficial soreness* this is virtually confined to the erupting lower third molar (wisdom tooth), although it may complicate eruption of the upper wisdom tooth also. It thus occurs at about 20 years of age and presents itself with acute pain, swelling noted over and beneath the angle of the mandible and severe trismus. Tender submandibular or upper cervical lymphadenopathy is the rule. Examination, which is admittedly *difficult,* reveals considerable inflammation with swelling and maceration of the gum in the lower third molar region. The wisdom tooth may not be visible but is at least palpable and pus can usually be expressed from around the operculum.

The upper third molar can usually be seen to be biting on the inflamed lower gum and this proves by far the most important initiating and aggravating factor in acute pericoronitis. X-rays, which have to be taken externally, show an erupting or impacted wisdom tooth.

Treatment consists of removal of opposing upper third molar, antibiotics, hot salt mouth baths and, in suitable cases, application of trichloracetic acid followed by glycerine to the pericoronal cleft.

An important clinical variant of acute pericoronitis is not uncommon, in which pus forms around the wisdom tooth and burrows forward at the depths of the buccal sulcus and becomes prominent as a swelling and 'points' adjacent to the corresponding first or second molar. In such cases the first or second molar is often removed in the mistaken belief that they are the origin of a dento-alveolar abscess and the focus of infection is left untreated to flare up again at a later date.

d. ACUTE POST-EXTRACTION OSTEITIS: This, of course, is characterized by occurring only after tooth extraction. The pain usually starts two days after extraction and becomes maximal after a further 48 hours. The pain is very severe, dull, gnawing, persistent, throbbing, and associated with foul taste in the mouth (cacogeusia). A dry socket takes about a fortnight to become symptom-free.

In a typical case, examination reveals an empty (hence dry) socket in which food debris has accumulated. The surrounding mucosa is inflamed and very tender, but any swelling is rare. Tender regional lymphadenopathy is the rule. The only trap for the unwary is to glance and observe that the socket appears healed. In fact, college tweezers may be slipped painlessly into the socket and on opening to separate overlying socket lips an empty socket is revealed.

The opposite trap is to dismiss all post-extraction pain as dry socket, when it may be another faulty tooth or a root in the socket. The symptoms must be correlated with the physical signs. X-rays usually reveal simply a socket, but occasionally a tooth will be identified or a piece of amalgam filling in the socket. These should be removed rapidly, as healing does not occur in their presence.

Washing out the socket reveals exposed bone which is not sensitive. Any loose or protruding pieces are removed and the socket packed with either zinc oxide and eugenol, Dentalone, acriflavine pack or a gauze pack soaked in Whitehead's varnish (Tinct. Benz. Co.). Such packs should be changed on the third day and two suffice to allow granulations to cover all exposed vital bone. Any necrotic bone is picked out and healing follows rapidly. In the rare case with persistent symptoms, surgery to remove necrotic bone and sequestra may be necessary. Antibiotics play no part in the management of dry socket.

e. ACUTE OSTEOMYELITIS: This usually follows extraction of a tooth, although it may arise from spread of periapical infection and is virtually confined to the mandible. Symptomatically, it resembles dry socket, though it is associated with swelling and involvement of the inferior dental neurovascular bundle hence mental anaesthesia.

Collections of pus form which superficially resemble dento-alveolar abscess and these break down to form sinuses. Involved teeth loosen. After 10 days or so the extent of sequestration becomes apparent on X-rays.

Treatment is by antibiotics followed by removal of sequestra with saucerization when localization is complete.

f. INFECTED DENTAL CYST: This may be *symptomatically indistinguishable* from a dento-alveolar abscess, but X-rays reveal the true nature of affairs. Proper management is to control the acute phase and subsequently treat the cyst surgically. In selected cases enucleation may be the treatment of choice for even infected cysts.

g. ACUTE MAXILLARY SINUSITIS: This disorder commonly follows a mild upper respiratory tract infection but may also arise from periapical infection of upper teeth, or more commonly is the mode of presentation of unnoticed oro-antral fistula, while the course of established untreated oro-antral fistula may be punctuated by recurrent sinusitis. The symptoms are characteristically those of acute inflammatory pain which is centred in the cheek and radiates to the ipsilateral supra-orbital region. Swelling here is manifested as unilateral nasal obstruction and mucopurulent rhinorrhea; *there is never any swelling of the face.* As previously mentioned, the pain may appear to originate in the upper teeth which, anyway, are often periostitic. The pain is characteristically worsened towards the evening and by bending forward and lying down. Confirmation may be obtained by transillumination of the antra and radiography with a 10° occipitomental film.

Treatment is by use of antibiotics and agents to promote mucosal shrinkage of which ½ per cent ephedrine nose drops and inhalation of Friars' balsam or menthol crystals are most efficacious.

h. ACUTE CERVICAL LYMPHADENITIS: This may be associated with any of the above lesions or others of the head and neck, such as tonsillitis, otitis and skin infections, but may also apparently occur de novo (*see* Chapter 4). Severe pain is unusual, tenderness more common, slight trismus may occur as movements of the jaw are painful, but is never more than minimal.

i. ACUTE SOFT-TISSUE INFECTIONS: By this is meant involvement of the tissue spaces about the jaw including a pre-suppurative phase and abscess formation. These two stages are difficult to distinguish, which fact influences management. These infections may arise from any of the preceding except maxillary sinusitis, but are a rare sequel to dry socket. The spaces involved are the submandibular, sublingual, submasseteric and lateral pharyngeal. The characteristic inflammatory pain is usually less severe in these cases, swelling being a more prominent symptom. The swelling is brawny and firm and overlying skin is reddened.

These infections require antibiotics and incision for drainage if there is suspicion of pus at first or if improvement does not occur in 48 hours. No heat should be applied to the skin over the affected area.

Dull pain: Pain presenting as a dull ache commonly causes the greatest difficulty in diagnosis. Pain due to local disease in the jaw may closely simulate that of atypical facial pain and temporomandibular joint dysarthrosis. It is most important to take a full history followed by careful clinical and complete *radiological examination* to exclude organic disease. The local causes of dull aching pain are legion; the following list covers the majority and they are arranged according to the radiological appearances, the X-ray being the most important investigation in such cases:

    a. Buried teeth and roots.
    b. No abnormality in the bone of the jaws.
        i. Chronic pulpitis, resorption of teeth.
        ii. Chronic maxillary sinusitis.
        iii. Carcinoma of the maxillary antrum.
        iv. Post-extraction 'neuralgias'.
    c. Radiolucency of the jaws.
        i. Periapical granuloma.
        ii. Dental cysts, periapical, dentigerous, residual and keratocysts.
        iii. Non-odentogenic cysts.
        iv. Ameloblastoma.
        v. Giant-cell granuloma.
        vi. Malignant tumours of the jaws.
        vii. Benign tumours of the jaws.
        viii. Central granulomas (histiocytosis).
    d. Radiopaque lesions.
        i. Odontomes.
        ii. Periapical osteofibromas (cementomas).
        iii. Fibrous dysplasia.
        iv. Osteomas, osteoid osteoma.
        v. Osteosarcomas.
        vi. Chronic osteomyelitis.
        vii. Paget's disease.
        viii. Sclerosing metastases.
        ix. Caffey's disease.
    e. Blood vessels.

a. Buried Teeth and Roots. These, by casting an unmistakable shadow on the X-ray, present little problem in diagnosis; the difficulty arises in assessing the significance of such shadows. It is unusual for completely buried teeth and roots without associated infection evidenced by localized radiolucency to cause any pain. Clinically, a sinus may be present and then no difficulty arises, but in its absence the decision to remove the tooth or roots will depend upon the severity of the pain and the personality of the patient. If it is felt that the patient is genuine, then the tooth or roots are removed but with the warning that pain may not be cured. Otherwise the patient may be reviewed in three or six months and the case re-assessed.

b. i. *Chronic Pulpitis:* This may cause dull pain and can be very difficult to diagnose. The causes basically are the same as for acute pulpitis (*see above*) and diagnostic methods are similar. Rarely idiopathic internal resorption of the pulp, which may be detected on the X-ray, will cause pain similar to that of chronic pulpitis. In either case extraction or root-canal therapy will be required.

ii *Chronic maxillary sinusitis* may prove difficult to diagnose and typical symptoms include mucopurulent nasal discharge and a feeling of fullness in the cheek. Suspicion should lead to an ENT consultation.

iii. *Carcinoma of the maxillary antrum* may lead to dull pain but other features will normally lead to a diagnosis.

iv. *Post-extraction 'neuralgias':* After extraction of teeth there may be localized dull pain exacerbated by pressure from a denture. This has been thought to be due to neuromas developing in torn pulpal nerve fibres. The pain may be relieved by curettage (rarely) but tend to remit spontaneously.

c. i. *Chronic Periapical Granulomas (or Small Cysts):* These are almost invariably painless but may cause pain. The associated teeth require removal, or root canal treatment.

ii–viii. Dental cysts are rarely painful and the same applies to non-odontogenic cysts, ameloblastomas and giant-cell granulomas. Malignant central tumours of the jaws (most usually metastases) are frequently painful as are histiocytomas. In this context are included leukaemic deposits and multiple myelomatosis. Benign central tumours of the jaws are the most rare of this group of central, radiolucent, space-occupying lesions and they are not commonly painful.

d. i. *Odontomes:* are not commonly painful and are usually readily distinguished from other radiopaque lesions on their radiographic appearance.

ii. *Periapical osteofibromas* which may be multiple, especially in Negroes, are an occasional cause of dull pain.

iii. *Fibrous dysplasia* is usually painless.

iv. *Osteomas of the jaws* are rare and usually painless but the even rarer osteoid osteoma may be the cause of considerable dull aching pain.

v. *Osteosarcoma* is usually a painful lesion; in the jaws it is almost always confined to the mandible. There may be considerable clinical and radiological difficulty in distinguishing it from chronic osteomyelitis. In either case, however, surgical exploration is advisable and histological examination of operative material provides the correct diagnosis.

vi. *Chronic osteomyelitis* provides a spectrum of radiological appearances from simple radiolucency to dense osteosclerosis. Sequestra may or may not be apparent. In children, frequently a very florid periosteal reaction may occur without suppuration (Garré's osteomyelitis). In most cases there is a severe dull aching pain.

vii. *Paget's disease,* which in the jaws is almost confined to the maxilla, is also associated with dull pain but the diagnosis is usually obvious as the skull and other bones are widely involved.

viii. *Sclerosing metastases* (including leukaemic deposits) are rare in the jaws but may cause severe pain.

ix. *Caffey's disease* is a rarity but causes pain in infants in the face and limbs. X-rays reveal subperiosteal new bone formation.

Temporomandibular joint and salivary gland diseases are considered in separate chapters later.

e. Blood Vessels: Giant-cell arteritis. Syn. Cranial arteritis, Temporal arteritis and including Polymyalgia rheumatica and Polymyalgia arteritica.

This disease of the aged is of unknown aetiology, although it certainly has many features of an auto-immune disorder.

Pathology

Although clinical features are usually due to disease of the superficial temporal arteries, or others of similar size in the head and neck, pathological examination reveals that many vessels may be involved in the disease, from the aorta onward. Occlusion of the lumina of large vessels exceptionally occurs and this disease may be the basis of Takayashu's (pulseless) disease.

The affected vessel shows destruction of the internal elastic lamina and proliferation of the intima but the principal changes are in the media with granulomatous inflammation and giant-cells which are specific to the condition. There is a chronic inflammatory infiltration around the vessel and the lumen is diminished or obliterated. The pathological basis of the characteristic arthropathy and muscle wasting in polymyalgia rheumatica is unknown, but its association is confirmed by the presence of the arteritis in the superficial temporal artery even in the absence of local symptoms.

Clinical features

The disease occurs after the age of 55 and is most common after the age of 70.

There is systemic upset characterized by fever, malaise, anorexia with leucocytosis and anaemia. Typically there is pain in one or both temples with tenderness of the associated scalp. The pain is dull and persistent and may be severe and the tenderness of the scalp prevents sleep. The pain may radiate into the face or occipital region and there may be ischaemic pain in the muscles of mastication on chewing. Examination reveals a thickened tortuous temporal artery which is pulseless (or becomes so). In up to half of the cases, blindness develops (which may be bilateral) and in a number of cases there are other ischaemic neurological syndromes. Rarely there may be gangrene of the scalp or tongue. The sedimentation rate is elevated, often strikingly so, due to hyperfibrinogenaemia. The diagnosis is established by biopsy of the affected vessel under local analgesia and this often has value in relieving local symptoms.

In the majority of cases the disease burns itself out in six months to two years. Steroids are vital as soon as the diagnosis is considered probable since they are of undoubted value in preventing the catastrophic ischaemic complications and in the meantime control the symptoms and improve the wellbeing of the patient. The dose is 60 mg of prednisone daily which is reduced after one month to a maintenance dose depending upon the ESR and symptoms and is withdrawn after six months to one year.

Referred Pain

a. Eye: The source of pain in eye lesions is usually obvious, the only possible exception being acute (closed angle) glaucoma. The pain is severe and may radiate across one side of the face. Vomiting may occur. Vision is rapidly lost in the affected eye which shows a dull, sea green, oval, dilated pupil through a misty cornea with circum-corneal vascular injection, the globe being stony hard.

b. Ear: Referred pain from the ear to the face is unusual. It is associated with other signs of ear disease such as deafness, vertigo, tinnitus and discharge. Conversely, however, pain in the ear referred from the teeth (or temporomandibular joint) is exceedingly common. The teeth usually at fault are lower molars, particularly the third.

c. Heart: Ischaemic pain derived from the myocardium may radiate into the mandible and rarely may occur there without associated central chest pain but there is usually concurrent pain in the elbow and wrist. The pain is precipitated by exercise, emotion and eating, and remits in a few minutes. Pain due to invasion of the superior mediastinum, usually by a bronchial carcinoma, may radiate into the jaws and face bilaterally. It is severe, constant and gnawing but obviously originates in the chest and is associated with superior vena caval obstruction.

d. Cervical Spine: Cervical spondylosis may be associated with pain radiating to the face, but facial pain alone is exceptionally, if ever, due to degenerative vertebral disease. Cervical spondylosis is associated with local pain which extends up over the occiput and corresponding root pain. Pain, if extending on to the face, is associated with pain in the neck, which is exacerbated by movement. X-rays usually reveal loss of intervertebral spaces and osteophytes.

e. *Oesophagus:* Pain from oesophageal disease may be referred to the lower jaw (and ear) but is associated with sialorrhoea and dysphagia.

Acknowledgement

Some of the material in this chapter was first published in *Dental Update*, May 1977 and is reproduced by kind permission of the publishers and editor.

Bibliography

Alestig K. and Barr J. (1963) Giant-cell arteritis. *Lancet* 1, 1228.

Alling C. C. (ed.) (1968) *Facial Pain*. Philadelphia, Lea & Febiger.

Hamrin B., Jonsson N. and Landberg T. (1965). Involvement of large vessels in polymyalgia arteritica. *Lancet* 1, 1193.

Meadows S. P. (1967) 'Giant-cell arteritis and blindness.' *Hosp. Med.* 1, 835.

Melzack R. and Wall P. D. (1965) Pain mechanisms, a new theory. *Science* 150, 971.

Merskey H. and Spear F. G. (1967) *Pain: Psychological and Psychiatric Aspects*. London, Baillière, Tindall and Cox.

Wyke, B. (1968), The neurology of facial pain. *Br. J. Hosp. Med.* 2, 46.

Chapter 16

Facial Pain. II. Diseases of the Temporomandibular Joint

Introduction

Lesions of this joint comprise arthritides of varied aetiology which are rare and a functional dysarthrosis which accounts for the majority of temporomandibular joint problem in dental practice. Since limitation of movement of the mandible is an important symptom of temporomandibular joint disease, a section on the causes of that is included.

They will be considered in the following order:

1. Temporomandibular dysarthrosis.
2. Temporomandibular arthritis.
3. Limitation of mandibular movement.

Temporomandibular Dysarthrosis

(Pain dysfunction syndrome; Costen's syndrome; temporomandibular joint syndrome; internal derangement; facial arthromyalgia).

Definition

A chronic disorder characterized by pain, clicking and trismus in the absence of radiographic or pathological abnormality, probably due to a functional derangement of the dental articulation.

Introduction

In 1934 Costen described the syndrome, which still bears his name, comprising facial neuralgia with otalgia and various otological symptoms which could be cured by occlusal equilibration, and he directed attention to the temporomandibular joint as the focal point of the syndrome. Costen attributed the symptoms to backward displacement of the condylar head with compression of the Eustachian tube and pressure upon the chorda tympani and auriculotemporal nerves.

The otological symptoms described by Costen included:
1. Continuous or intermittent deafness.
2. Stuffy sensation in the ears.
3. Tinnitus.
4. Dizziness (vertigo).

The pain, apart from otalgia, he described as neuralgia extending to the vertex, the occiput and temporal area ('sinus symptoms') with burning sensations of the tongue, nose and throat. He also described pain in the temporomandibular joint, clicking, trismus and the importance of disordered occlusion (he stressed overclosure).

Although Costen did a valuable service in recognizing the importance of temporomandibular dysarthrosis in the aetiology of facial pain and the basic importance of the dental occlusion in the aetiology of dysarthrosis, he probably cast the net too wide, and there is no doubt that very few, if any, patients have any otological or other bizarre symptoms attributable to joint dysfunction. Since the present use of the temporomandibular joint dysfunction implies something quite different from that envisaged by Costen, the eponymous title for the syndrome is best avoided.

Aetiology and pathogenesis

The condyle itself is not a weight-bearing joint; the occlusal surfaces of the teeth subserving this function with the oral cavity as the 'joint cavity'. The mandible is thus unique in possessing three 'joint' surfaces, one of which bears weight and frequently contains foreign bodies in the shape of food, pipes (the occlusal surfaces of the teeth) and other objects.

The condylar heads have to accommodate themselves in the glenoid fossae and the whole movement of the mandible is integrated by proprioceptive feedback from the muscles, the periodontal membranes of the teeth and the capsule of the joint. High restorations in the teeth may lead to avoiding action by the mandible leading to the bite of convenience with 'condylar displacement', as may one or more teeth in malocclusion. Erupting wisdom teeth or other painful teeth may lead to bites of convenience. The syndrome also occurs in patients with a normal occlusion and may be due simply to excessive and abnormal condylar movements.

With loss of the teeth and their replacement by prostheses, the possibilities of the development of joint dysfunction are enhanced. Condylar displacement may be due to incorrect recording of the bite or later by progressive wear of the occlusal surfaces.

In this context 'condylar displacement' implies that the dental articulation (the overriding influence) can only be achieved at the expense of some continuous muscle activity ('spasm') or abnormal posture of the muscles. Pain may then be due to pressure on the posterior third of the inter-articular disc, but most of the symptoms are attributable to excessive or incoordinate muscle activity, which is itself protective in that it maintains the occluding surfaces of the teeth at the expense of one or, more rarely, both temporomandibular joints.

There is no set pattern of occlusal dysharmony consistently associated with dysarthrosis and many patients are seen with gross malocclusion or loss of molar support who do not develop joint symptoms. Conversely, however, occlusal factors are directly remediable and there is no doubt as to the remission of symptoms following correction of occlusal abnormalities in some cases. There must be another conditioning factor which operates in the patients who develop the syndrome and this may lie in the personality. There is growing evidence that in many cases 'stress' may be significant while in many cases depressive symptoms are present. There is an extensive literature on the relationship between this disorder, personality, neuroticism and anxiety/depression which is somewhat inconclusive. This, probably, is due to the inadequacy of current investigative and psychometric techniques. It is undoubted that many of the patients are somewhat introspective worriers and 'suffer' from disorders which their more phlegmatic brethren pass off as a transient nuisance only. They also suffer more frequently than the general population from migraine and musculoskeletal troubles such as 'fibrositis,' backache and headache. Anstie, writing on neuralgia in 1871, said of a group of diseases called 'myalgia', which would undoubtedly include this syndrome, that 'It is essentially pain produced in a muscle obliged to work when its structure is imperfectly nourished or impaired by disease'. He also noted the following points in the differential diagnosis from 'neuralgia':

'Attacks a limited patch, or patches, that can be identified with the tendon or aponeurosis of a muscle which, in inquiry, will be found to have been hardly worked.'

'As often as not occurs in persons with no special neurotic tendency.'

'Is inevitably and very severely aggravated by every movement of the part.'

'Distinguished, from the first, by local tenderness on pressure as well as on movement.'

'Tender points correspond to tendinous origins and insertions of muscles.'

'Pain usually completely, and always considerably, relieved by full extension of the painful muscle or muscles.'

Bruxism is the habit of tooth-grinding or clenching, due to anxiety, which may be an important initiating or aggravating factor but in my experience rarely very significant. It may occur at night (some authorities call this bruxomania) and is then frequently expressed as joint stiffness or pain over the muscles of mastication on wakening. In such cases the teeth often show marked wear facets. The temporomandibular joints suffer, as does the spouse!

The *pathology* of temporomandibular dysarthrosis is unknown since the disorder is benign and essentially self-limited so that pathological material is not available. The temporomandibular joint disc has been removed not infrequently for otherwise incurable dysarthrosis and has been shown to be the seat of neo-vascularization, degeneration and calcification.

Clinical features

The patients are more frequently female and all ages are represented between 15 years and old age, but there is a sharp peak incidence in the early twenties.

The cardinal symptoms are:
1. Pain.
2. Trismus (limitation of movement of the mandible due to muscle spasm), and episodes of joint locking.
3. Clicking joint.

These three symptoms are present usually for at least six months, but often for many years, before the patient presents and there is some fluctuation in their severity; not all three need be present but it would be very difficult to sustain the diagnosis on the basis of one symptom alone.

1. *Pain:* The pain is a dull ache which may be limited to the region of the joint but may radiate to the temple or down over the ascending ramus of the mandible and frequently behind the ear. Occasionally the pain is felt purely as an otalgia (earache). In this variety there are no other features of ear disease—deafness, tinnitus or discharge—and examination of the drum shows no abnormality.

The pain is characteristically made worse by movement of the jaw and particularly chewing, which may lead to sharp pain radiating widely.

Occasionally the pain is of a neuralgic quality that is rather shooting and confined to the territory of a peripheral nerve. This is frequently the auriculotemporal nerve, but may be maxillary or mandibular division of the trigeminal; such a pain may extend into the tongue.

2. *Trismus:* This varies in degree and in the most severe cases opening is limited to about 15 mm, but incisor separation usually is less severely restricted; in at least a third of the cases trismus is absent, but there is a history of previous episodes of limited opening. Since the limitation is frequently unilateral, it leads to deviation of the jaw on opening towards the affected side, but this is not invariable even with strictly unilateral disease. The trismus is often worst in the morning on awakening, which may be an indication of bruxism. Alternatively, the 'stiffness' of the jaw may worsen progressively as the day advances. The limitation is functional as can be assessed from the history in which the patient describes the limitation as varying. Also the mouth may be *passively* opened to full extent by gentle finger pressure on the lower incisors. This is only slightly painful and demonstrates that ankylosis is not present. Under anaesthesia, of course, mouth opening is normal. Restriction of anterior movement of the condyle is demonstrated by lack of lateral movement of the mandible to the opposite side with the teeth slightly separated.

Episodes of locking are characteristic of the syndrome. In these the mandible becomes immobile usually in the half to three-quarters open position. Such locking is transient and most patients are able to manipulate the joint to normal movement. In a few the locking is persistent and such cases may be referred to, quite mistakenly, as subluxation of the joint (*see* p. 208).

3. *Click:* This is a common symptom and may precede development of pain and trismus by months or years. The loudest clicks are audible to the observer unaided, but all can be heard with a stethoscope.

The click usually only occurs with the incisors *separated by a few millimetres,* as the condyle starts its translatory movement in the lower joint compartment. It also occurs at the corresponding point in closure of the jaw. Rarely, the click may occur at the end of opening or before the jaw is fully open. The click has been said to be due to an abnormal relationship between the condyle and the articular disc. The early click is adduced as evidence of posterior displacement of the condyle so that the disc lies in front instead of above it, so that on opening the condyle snaps into its proper position and redisplaces at the end of closure. The click at the end of opening is said to be due to slipping of the condyle past the anterior end of the disc, but it is doubtful if either simple structural explanation is reasonable.

It is more likely that the click originates in muscle imbalance with sudden recruitment, thus the noise. A click without any other symptoms is very common and the patient should be reassured that it is of no significance.

Other symptoms: Otological symptoms, as described by Costen, seem to occur quite infrequently.

Examination must include:

   1. The joint.
   2. The muscles.
   3. The teeth: (*a*) general examination for other sources of pain; (*b*) occlusion.

1. *The Joint:* The joint should be palpated to elicit tenderness, without which the diagnosis is hardly tenable, and the patient asked to move the jaw to the fullest extent so that the movement of each condyle may be ascertained; this is most readily done from behind the patient. The degree of *movement* may be best assessed by observing the movements of the mandible from the front. The examination should start with the teeth in occlusion and the freeway space is assessed; it should not exceed 5 mm.

The mouth should then be opened as widely as possible and the amount of opening measured between the upper and lower central incisors. Most patients with this syndrome open the mouth with irregular slight deviations from side to side which are highly characteristic.

Finally, with the teeth just parted, the lateral excursion of the mandible to each side is measured.

2. *The muscles:* These should be carefully palpated to elicit tenderness and spasm. The pterygoid sign is a pathognomic physical sign in this syndrome. It is the marked tenderness of the origin of lateral pterygoid as palpated above and behind the maxillary tuberosity.

3. *The teeth:* These should be examined *individually* for caries, restorative work (especially recent) and the presence of periostitic teeth. In younger patients erupting wisdom teeth should be carefully noted, and any tenderness in their vicinity. The overall wear of the occlusal surfaces of the teeth should be noted; highly polished facets on fillings are particularly significant. Dentures should be examined for fit and stability.

The jaw relationship should be recorded and the position of occlusion, and the patient instructed to close from the rest position until any tooth contact occurs. The point or points of contact are noted, and the patient instructed to then close fully. This establishes the presence of premature contacts and subsequent cuspal guidance to an eccentric bite. Wax wafers or articulating paper may be useful in this part of the examination which is extremely important and often time-consuming.

Finally, models of the teeth from alginate impressions are prepared and articulated in the position of initial contact; the models can then be ground in to the centric occlusion, which should confirm the clinical examination.

Radiography

This is invariably carried out and characteristically fails to show any abnormality in the articulating surfaces of the joint. Narrowing of the joint space and posterior displacement of the condyle may be seen, but radiography is so routinely unrewarding that it might be worth avoiding if the diagnosis is obvious.

Diagnosis is usually straightforward but it is important that all other possible causes of pain in the teeth are eliminated before the dysarthrosis is treated.

Treatment

Explanation and reassurance are the first and most important parts of treatment. It is necessary to explain the muscular nature of symptoms, their benignity, and the fact that arthritis does not supervene. Consideration should be given to the patient's home circumstances, job, immediate relatives, finance and other worries. Depressed patients should be given either amitriptyline or prothiaden (75 mg nocte), while in anxiety diazepam or chlordiazepoxide 10 mg nocte.

In a small number of cases with severe pain and marked trismus a short course of oxyphenbutazone (100–200 mg tds) or similar drug is very useful.

High fillings are polished or replaced. Interfering cusps are ground to balance the occlusion. Painful teeth are dealt with and where erupting wisdom teeth are thought to be an aggravating factor, arrangements made to remove them.

Cases where there is severe loss of posterior support simply require dental care including dentures. In the edentulous, new dentures restoring the correct occlusal height are indicated.

In the many cases with no obvious local cause, which includes the bulk of young patients, a simple upper bite-raising appliance is both diagnostic and can be used as the main therapeutic measure. It is constructed of a simple acrylic plate with Adam's cribs on the molars and a flat anterior bite-plane designed to open the bite about 3–4 mm (bringing the incisors almost to an edge-to-edge relationship).

This plate should be worn continuously and symptoms almost completely remit in about a fortnight with its use. At this stage, it is prudent to recheck the occlusion since irregularities may now be revealed, the plate having broken an acquired avoidance reflex which disguised the occlusal discrepancy at the first visit. As soon as symptoms have remitted, the plate may be worn at night only and then discarded in six months, when in the majority of cases the symptoms do not recur. Alternatively, a vacuum-formed lower splint in soft acrylic is equally effective.

In cases in which there appears to be overclosure, especially the Class II, division 2, cases, or those associated with bruxism, relief of symptoms may demand a metal overlay denture which itself may have to be preceded by the crowning of several teeth.

Intra-articular injection of steroids and short-wave diathermy are mentioned only to condemn them.

Surgery has a debatable role. It is advocated in the quite exceptional patient in whom the dysfunction is related to posturing associated with jaw deformities. The surgery is then directed to the primary abnormality. Surgery of the joint itself is hard to justify but is advocated by some for cases in which conservative management fails. Meniscectomy has been discarded and replaced by condylar shave (high partial condylectomy) or, more frequently, condylotomy (osteotomy of the condylar neck with subsequent spontaneous union). Unfortunately the place of operation and its value remain shrouded in mystery (as is true with most aspects of this disorder).

Temporomandibular Arthritis

1. Suppurative:
   i. Spread from contiguous structures
      a. Mastoid
      b. Mandible   } Streptococcal.
      c. Overlying skin and parotid

   ii. Haematogenous   Staphylococcal.
                                    Streptococcal.
                                    Gonococcal.

2. Tuberculous.
3. Rheumatoid disease.
4. Osteoarthrosis.
5. Gout.
6. Traumatic.

1. *Acute suppurative arthritis* of the mandibular joint is a rarity and has become more so since the introduction of antibiotics which effectively control otitis media, previously the commonest source of the infection. Infection may rarely spread up from ascending ramus of the mandible affected by osteomyelitis and exceptionally may reach the joint from the overlying skin or parotid gland. Haematogenous arthritis may occur during the course of scarlatina (*S. pyogenes*), staphylococcal septicaemia and gonorrhoea.

Pathology: The joint cavity is filled with pus and the adjacent cartilage and bone destroyed. In the untreated case there is progression to complete bony ankylosis but effective treatment may produce a complete return to normality or minimal fibrous ankylosis.

Clinically: The patient presents with severe pain, local swelling and marked trismus. These may simulate acute parotitis or submasseteric abscess.

Treatment with antibiotics is indicated and incision for drainage if early resolution does not occur. Later, when the acute stage is passed, active jaw exercises are required.

2. *Tuberculous and syphilitic arthritis* are extreme rarities.

3. *Rheumatoid disease* attacks the temporomandibular joint in about a quarter of all cases in which the disease assumes a severe and progressive nature. It is unusual in patients only mildly afflicted. Pain is not usually severe and limitation of opening is the common mode of presentation. The condylar head may be progressively eroded away until the stump of the condylar neck 'articulates' via a mobile fibrous ankylosis with the glenoid fossa.

Diagnosis is usually straightforward since the hallmarks of rheumatoid disease are evident all over the patient. No specific local treatment is indicated, although severe limitation of movement demands condylectomy.

Juvenile rheumatoid arthritis (Still's disease) may cause a similar severe arthritis in childhood in which the problem of ankylosis is compounded by that of mandibular hypoplasia due to cessation of mandibular growth.

4. *Osteoarthrosis* is a degenerative disorder which has a very high asymptomatic incidence in all joints after middle age, and the temporomandibular joint is no exception. It is unusual, however, to see a

patient with osteoarthrosis causing the typical symptoms of painful limitation of movement with crepitus with radiological findings to support the diagnosis, namely loss of joint space, osteosclerosis of joint surfaces and osteophytes.

If analgesics fail to allow proper function, condylotomy or condylectomy may be advisable, but should be avoided as it seems that the majority of patients become pain free with an adequate range of movements during the course of a year or two. This happy outcome may be facilitated by intra-articular hydrocortisone during the acute phase.

5. *Gouty arthritis* is rare in the temporomandibular joint, occurring only in advanced cases.

6. *Traumatic*. This is not an arthritis in the accepted sense, but some local inflammation may occur due to damage of tissues and haemarthrosis may be present. It is, of course, due to *indirect* trauma to the joint transmitted by a blow to the mandible with the teeth apart.

Trismus is marked and rest leads to resolution.

Limitation of Mandibular Movement

This is an extremely common symptom and may be due to either:
1. Trismus—Muscle spasm.
2. Ankylosis—Organic or structural limitation of condylar movement.

Such ankylosis may be intra-articular or extra-articular.

1. *Trismus*

Trismus is itself a symptom and has several causes which are subdivisible into three groups. There are those due to painful *acute inflammatory disease* around the ascending ramus of the mandible. Diagnosis is effected from the associated features of the underlying disease. The second group of disorders are due to direct *injury* to or *inflammation* of the *masticatory muscles* themselves and the third—of which trismus is only an incidental and unimportant feature—are due to disorders of the *central nervous system*.

Acute inflammatory disease: The majority of cases are due to local inflammatory disease which includes pericoronitis of upper and lower wisdom teeth, dento-alveolar abscesses on wisdom teeth, temporomandibular arthritis, acute tonsillitis, quinsy, parotitis and otitis externa, and complete trismus is usual with tissue space infections around the ascending ramus of the jaw, namely submasseteric abscess or pharyngeal abscess, or in the temporal fossa or pterygopalatine fossa. In these cases the trismus is usually severe and develops rapidly. There is local pain and swelling and the usual signs of an inflammatory process. Trismus is rare or only slight in cases of cervical lymphadenitis, however acute. Trismus is *also* a feature of fractured mandible when it may then be due to pain on movement of the mandible, but in injuries of the temporomandibular joint a mechanical element is added as is the case in fractures of the zygoma and zygomatic arch. Dislocation of the head of the condyle also accounts for limitation of opening, as may direct trauma to the muscles of mastication.

Trismus is to be expected after operations involving the jaws and tends to remit slowly during the subsequent 10 days. Its degree can be minimized by gentle handling. Greenfield and Moore (1969) have shown that the trismus is not due to masticatory muscle activity antagonizing movement of the mandible but rather an inhibition of all muscle activity connected with the mandible, including the inframandibular muscles, and this inhibition also prevents forceful biting of the jaws in which elevators and depressors of the mandible normally act synergistically.

In all these cases the trismus remits with treatment of the underlying disorder and relaxes if a general anaesthetic is given.

Diseases or inflammation of the muscles: As mentioned above, direct trauma to the muscles, which may be operative, causes trismus. A common variety is that due to trauma from a needle used for an inferior dental block and rarely this is followed by fibrous ankylosis (*see below*).

Postoperative trismus and that due to direct trauma to muscles *always remits entirely in 3 weeks* (more commonly within 1 week).

Direct invasion of muscles by local carcinoma may lead to trismus (characteristically by nasopharyngeal carcinoma as part of Trotter's syndrome). Trichinosis during the actue invasive stage may be associated with trismus but is very rare. Trismus may be a feature of dystrophia myotonica or myotonia congenita.

Central Causes: Involvement of the trigeminal nerve or its central connections.

a. Tetanus is characteristically associated with trismus which is spasmodic, painful and associated with progressive involvement of other muscle groups.

b. Rabies may cause trismus but there is extensive spasm of pharyngeal muscles.

c. Trismus may occur in tetany but then follows carpopedal spasm and tingling sensation in the hands and around the mouth.

d. Trismus is a feature, albeit minor, of strychnine poisoning.

e. Trismus may occur in widespread brain damage as in encephalitis or in lesions involving the upper motor neurones such as cerebral space occupying lesion, but again is not a presenting symptom, the trismus being a minor component of the illness.

f. Trismus associated with other facial spasms may occur in idiopathic dyskinesia (facial hemispasm), and a similar syndrome may be produced by phenothiazine drugs.

g. Hysteria and malingering are two causes of trismus of which malingering is rather more common and usually follows a genuine trismus. The malingerer may be caught out by sharp stimulation of the soft palate which causes gagging and wide-opening which the patient should observe in a mirror.

The hysterical patient may be treated in the same way, but allowance made for the fact that gagging may not occur with palatal stimulation in hysterics. The mouth may then be opened under anaesthesia and the opening demonstrated to the patient on waking.

2. Ankylosis

Intra-articular: Bony or fibrous ankylosis may follow trauma, acute suppurative arthritis or rheumatoid disease. In such cases the limitation of opening is usually marked, painless and present for a long time.

If occurring in childhood there may be associated condylar hypoplasia with characteristic mandibular deformity.

Extra-articular ankylosis: This may be produced by fibrous or bony connection between the mandible and the skull outside the joint capsule, or to scarring about the face produced by burns or trauma (operative or otherwise) or chronic infection.

Intra-oral scar bands may be due to operations and in Indians may be due to submucous fibrosis. It has also been reported following the ulceration of epidermolysis bullosa (Sowray and Rowe, 1965).

Scar bands may on occasion be stretched by progressive exercises but may require to be forcefully broken down under general anaesthesia or, in selected cases, excision may be advisable.

Fibrosis in the muscles of mastication may follow needle trauma as previously mentioned. Occasionally, following inferior dental nerve block, a localized fibrosis occurs in the medial pterygoid, presumably due to an organized haematoma, and this produces a typical limitation of opening. The patient can open freely to 10–15 mm when the movement is painlessly arrested, and attempts to move the mandible cause pain on the side of an inferior dental block given a fortnight to six weeks before. Such cases require forceful opening under general anaesthesia followed by exercises to maintain mobility.

Mechanical limitation of opening may occur in depressed fracture of the zygoma or zygomatic arch where these bones impinge upon the moving coronoid process.

After trauma a cause of prolonged trismus is the rare myositis ossificans in which the masseter or medial pterygoid may be involved.

Exceptionally, local bone excesses may lead to limitation of opening—they may be bony tumours of the ascending ramus of the jaw especially near the condyle, or the non-neoplastic coronoid hyperplasia (Rowe, 1963).

All these mechanical ankyloses require operative treatment.

In all cases in which a patient presents with limited opening of the mouth the opinion of an oral surgeon should be sought.

Chronic subluxation of both temporomandibular joints may occur following extraction of the teeth under general anaesthesia or in psychiatric patients. Initially the subluxation is maintained by spasm, but fibrosis ensues as the position may be maintained for months or years. This is distinguished from all other cases of limited opening since the jaw is partly open, and clinical and radiographic examination reveals that the condyle is not in the glenoid fossa, but in front of the eminentia articularis.

'Recurrent subluxation' is the name applied to the syndrome in which the head of the condyle is held, by elevator muscle activity, in front of the glenoid eminence, with the mouth widely open. It should be noted that this position is a normal one for the head of the condyle and so dislocation it is not. This syndrome is similar to 'locking' in temporomandibular joint dysfunction and may be closely simulated by the extrapyramidal side-effects of phenothiazines.

It occurs in the mentally retarded, psychiatric patients, following head and jaw injury and rarely in the myopathies. It also occurs in people who can at the best be regarded as stupid. The luxation is reduced by asking the patient to *open* against resistance followed by downward and backward pressure over the external oblique ridges of the mandible. In resistant cases intravenous diazepam (20 mg) improves the likelihood of success.

Bibliography

Banks P. and Mackenzie I. (1975) Condylotomy, a clinical and experimental appraisal. *Eur. J. Maxillofacial Surg.* **3**, 170.

Beekius G. J. and Harrington R. (1965) Trismus, its aetiology and management of difficulty in opening the mouth. *Laryngoscope* **75**, 1234.

Blackwood H. J. J. (1963) Arthritis of the mandibular joint. *Br. Dent. J.* **115**, 317.

Campbell W. (1965) Clinical radiological investigations of the mandibular joints. *Br. J. Radiol.* **38**, 401.

Costen J. B. (1951) The present status of the mandibular joint syndrome in otolaryngology. *Trans. Am. Acad. Ophthal.* **56**, 809

Franks A. S. T. (1965) Conservative treatment of temporomandibular joint dysfunction. *Dent. Pract.* **15**, 205.

Greenfield B. E. and Moore J. R. (1969) Electromyographic study of post-operative trismus. *J. Oral Surg.* **27**, 92.

Hankey G. T. (1954) Temporomandibular arthrosis. *Br. Dent. J.* **96**, 249.

Hankey G. T. (1958) Some observations on Costen's mandibular syndrome. *Proc. R. Soc. Med.* **51**, 225.

Lupton D. E. and Johnson D. L. (1973) Myofascial pain-dysfunction syndrome: Attitudes and other personality characteristics related to tolerance for pain. *J. Prosthet. Dent.* **29**, 323.

Rothwell P. S. (1972) Personality and temporomandibular joint dysfunction. *Oral Surg.* **34**, 734.

Rowe N. L. (1963) Bilateral developmental hyperplasia of the mandibular coronoid process. *Br. J. Oral Surg.* **1**, 90.

Sowray J. H. and Rowe N. L. (1965) Extra-articular ankylosis as a complication of dystrophic epidermolysis bullosa. *Br. J. Oral Surg.* **3**, 136.

Chapter 17

Facial Pain. III. Neuralgias

Paroxysmal Trigeminal Neuralgias

Definition

A sharp, severe paroxysmal pain of unknown aetiology occurring in the distribution of the trigeminal nerve.

Introduction

Avicenna (980–1037), the Arabian philosopher and physician, mentions this condition in *Canon of Medicine*. Trousseau (1801–1867), the French physician, thought with some justification that this condition had the character of a sensory epilepsy, hence the name he gave to it, 'neuralgie epileptiforme'.

It is not pure semantics to insist on the condition being called *paroxysmal* trigeminal neuralgia, as any facial pain is a trigeminal neuralgia (in one sense) but only this condition has paroxysmal character. To be very precise one should use the term 'idiopathic paroxysmal trigeminal neuralgia' to distinguish it from symptomatic trigeminal neuralgia, for which a cause can be found. Suffice to limit the terms to paroxysmal trigeminal neuralgia ('idiopathic' understood) and symptomatic paroxysmal neuralgia.

Aetiology

The cause seems to be a neurological short-circuiting which would appear to occur in the nerve roots and the Gasserian ganglion.

The concept of paroxysmal trigeminal neuralgia as being a sensory epilepsy does not seem to have any foundation if the lesion is peripheral but in fact the condition is more akin to epilepsy than any other. There are still many facets of this disease which are unexplained, among which remains the reason why it tends to remit and recur.

Clinical features

Twice as common in females as it is in males, paroxysmal trigeminal neuralgia is rare before the age of 40 and is most commonly seen in the age group 50–70 years. By far the majority of cases are unilateral, being slightly more common on the right than on the left. Harris, in his large series of over 2000 cases, described 6 per cent of cases as being bilateral. Most other authors put the figure much lower and one wonders if the great reputation of Harris attracted the bilateral cases where lesser men might try to treat the unilateral cases.

The pain is usually experienced in the second or third divisions of the trigeminal nerve, but rarely in the first division. It may be diffuse between these two divisions or it may be specific to the terminal branches of the nerve, e.g. being confined to the lingual or mental branches of the mandibular nerve.

The character of the pain is the diagnostic feature, usually being described as sharp and shooting 'like an electric shock' or a 'red-hot needle'. Each paroxysm of pain lasts only for a few seconds, but it may seem much longer to the patient. There are few more severe pains which afflict mankind and most patients will distort their faces and do anything for relief. Paroxysms are more common first thing in the morning and may follow each other in close succession. For some reason they are not so common at night. No doubt this repetitive feature has a psychological effect on the patient like the repetitive nature of uterine contractions in labour, or torture which has been planned with sadistic forethought.

Between paroxsyms the patient may not be completely pain-free; there may be a dull background ache. Status paroxysmal trigeminal neuralgia is fortunately very rare.

'Triggering' is another characteristic feature of this condition. There are certain areas of the face which if lightly stimulated will precipitate a paroxysm. The patient may describe acts of washing, shaving, eating or cleaning the teeth as initiating the pain. On occasions even talking, a draught on the face or the vibration of walking may cause a paroxysm. Paradoxically, the patient may touch the trigger area to show where it is without pain. In many cases the trigger area appears to be refractory between paroxysms, but there are rare cases in which the patient is afraid to wash or shave half the face.

There is a periodicity about the paroxysms: a number occur at frequent intervals and then the patient may be pain-free for weeks or even months before the condition occurs again. Each bout varies in its severity, as does the whole condition.

Physical examination

This should be complete, both local and general; any neurological abnormality other than a trigger zone should put the diagnosis of paroxysmal trigeminal neuralgia in doubt.

Course

It is well to remember, when making evaluation of any treatment, that the condition has natural remissions. Even when a bout has remitted, there is no way of predicting when or if another bout will occur, nor is there any way of telling what the severity will be. Suicides in untreated severe cases have been known.

Differential diagnosis

As the diagnosis is made almost totally from the history, every effort must be made to get an accurate history. Patients who give an over-dramatic account of facial pain with the use of superlatives to describe its features may be diagnosed as paroxysmal trigeminal neuralgia by the unwary. Conversely, there are stoical patients who play down the severity of their symptoms with the possible danger of a missed diagnosis. This may also occur if the patient has linguistic difficulties in describing his condition.

Dental causes of pain should be excluded. Exposed dentine can give a very sharp pain when it is stimulated. Any possible odontological cause should be treated, as its presence will only lead to confusion later, when the patient is under treatment for paroxysmal trigeminal neuralgia. In edentulous patients the mental nerve may be near the summit of the alveolar ridge, and pressure on it from the denture can cause a shooting pain that is not unlike paroxysmal trigeminal neuralgia.

Symptomatic Trigeminal Neuralgia: Any lesion pressing on the trigeminal nerve along its course can give paroxysmal pain which may be called symptomatic paroxysmal trigeminal neuralgia to distinguish it from idiopathic trigeminal neuralgia. The most common are lesions of the cerebellopontine angle, e.g. arterial aneurysms, acoustic neuromas and meningiomas. Compression of the trigeminal nerve branches in bony canals can also cause paroxysmal pain, as with Paget's disease of bone or acromegaly. All these causes are rare compared with idiopathic paroxysmal trigeminal neuralgia. A cholesteatoma of the ear may become extremely large, erode bone and eventually press on the trigeminal nerve root. Meningiomas of the trigeminal nerve are extremely rare, but it is uncommon even among these cases for the pain to be paroxysmal. Herpes zoster may give paroxysmal pain, but the cutaneous lesions make the diagnosis clear. If paroxysmal trigeminal neuralgia occurs with hemifacial spasm a lesion compressing both the fifth and seventh cranial nerves should be suspected.

Paroxysmal Trigeminal Neuralgia and Disseminated Sclerosis: According to Harris, 3·6 per cent of patients presenting as paroxysmal trigeminal neuralgia are, in fact, suffering from disseminated sclerosis. This should be suspected in all such patients below the age of 50 years, especially if the pain is in the first division of the nerve. This is yet another reason why all patients should undergo a full neurological examination.

Treatment

Many remedies have been tried in the desperate search to find an effective medical treatment. Many false hopes and claims have arisen as a result of the disease passing into a natural remission coincidentally with a specific remedy. One of the characteristics of paroxysmal trigeminal neuralgia is that it is not relieved by any of the standard analgesics. Of the many old remedies, the only one worth mentioning is *Gower's Mixture,* of which the active principle is tincture of gelsemium, an extract from the root of the yellow jasmine. It may be prescribed as follows and may be effective in minor cases:

tincture gelsemium	0·6 ml
glycerine trinitrate solution	0·1 ml
dilute hydrobromic acid	0·3 ml
tincture nux vomica	0·3 ml
lemon syrup	4·0 ml
add water to	15·0 ml

15 ml (one tablespoonful) should be taken 3 times a day.

If one is going to prescribe this rather old-fashioned mixture, it is as well to write the prescription in full, as there are four different Gower's mixtures in use.

Phenytoin sodium 100 mg tds has proved effective in some cases, but a patient can be admitted to hospital having taken an overdose of this drug in an attempt to gain relief from the pain.

Carbamazepine (Tegretol) provides the only effective medical treatment to date. This drug is a tricyclic compound very similar chemically to the antidepressant imipramine. It was discovered by Schindler of the Geigy Laboratories in 1953 as an anticonvulsant, but its potential in the treatment of paroxysmal trigeminal neuralgia was not realized until 1962, when Blom undertook the first clinical trial. Acting subthalamically between the trigeminal nucleus and the thalamus, possibly blocking synaptic conduction or enhancing reticular system inhibitor activity, it appears to give complete relief in over 50 per cent of cases and up to 90 per cent of patients get appreciable relief, although many may relapse. The great disadvantage of this drug is that over 60 per cent of patients suffer side effects. In the majority of patients these are minor and transient, giving ataxia, vertigo, drowsiness and gastrointestinal upsets which do not prevent continuation of therapy unless they become very severe. Old people may find the ataxia and vertigo disabling. All patients should be warned of these side effects, especially if they are in an occupation where they might be a danger to themselves or other people. A hypersensitivity type of maculopapular rash forbids further treatment with this drug. Cases of carbamazepine-induced cholestatic jaundice, discoid lupus erythematosus and erythema multiforme major (Stevens–Johnson syndrome) have been recorded. Three fatal cases of aplastic anaemia stand as a warning to all who prescribe this drug to monitor the patient's white cell count carefully and suspend therapy if it should fall below 3000 per c mm. Although no teratogenic side effects have yet been recorded, the drug should not be given in pregnancy.

Patients should be started on small doses, such as 100 mg (half a tablet) twice a day. This can be increased every 48 hours until an effective dose is found. Usually this is about 200 mg three or four times a day. Doses of 1·0 g or 1·2 g per day may be needed, but if these are not effective the patient should be referred for injection or surgery of the nerve. Although the manufacturers state that it is safe to give up to 1·6 g per day, there is little to be gained with these higher doses.

No patient should be left permanently on carbamazepine and all should be maintained on the minimal dose, so that the drug is gradually withdrawn. Recurrences are common with this mode of treatment and the drug becomes less effective as the condition progresses. Patients may easily become psychologically dependant on tablets for paroxysmal trigeminal neuralgia, even when they are getting little in the way of symptoms. It is recommended that carbamazepine be replaced gradually by chlordiazepoxide (Librium) in these doubtful cases: if the patient still remains pain-free he is no longer suffering from paroxysmal trigeminal neuralgia.

Phenytoin sodium (epanutin) up to 100 mg tds has a useful role as a second-line drug in cases which do not respond to carbamazepine or in whom carbamazepine has to be kept to low dosage because of side-effects.

Injection of local anaesthetic into the trigger area is a simple procedure which can be used to cover the period before carbamazepine becomes effective (carbamazepine may be effective very quickly, in as little as 48 hours). The remission of symptoms seems to be longer than the duration of the anaesthetic. If 2 per cent lignocaine is used it would be necessary to give two such injections per day. On these grounds it would seem logical to use a longer-acting local anaesthetic and amethocaine (Marcain) 0·5 per cent is useful as it is effective up to 24 hours.

Injection of alcohol into the ganglion is a great art which is safe only in the hands of the select few. X-ray control may be necessary to check the position of the needle before the injection is given. In the hands of the masters this is a good treatment. Relief may be gained for a period ranging from a few months to an average of eighteen months or two years, with a fair number of patients remaining pain-free indefinitely.

Surgical procedures: Peripheral neurolysis or neurectomy. When drugs fail or produce disabling side-effects and local anaesthesia of a peripheral branch of the trigeminal nerve produces remission, then neurolysis or neurectomy of that branch may be considered.

Neurolysis may be achieved by injection of alcohol (absolute) or phenol (5 per cent) or by cryoprobe (after surgical exposure). Neurectomy may be performed for the infraorbital, mental or inferior dental nerves. With more extensive involvement section of selected tracts in the nerve root or ganglion or section of the medullary tract may be indicated and for that neurosurgical opinion should be sought. The aim is to be selective in the area of anaesthesia, especially sparing the corneal reflex if at all possible. One warning with all patients submitted to surgery is to make sure by means of local anaesthesia that the patient knows what sensation he will lack in his face postoperatively. There are a few patients who would rather have the pain; one is tempted to think that their 'paroxysmal trigeminal neuralgia' is not of the severe type. Cases of atypical facial pain which have been submitted to this procedure still retain their pain, even though they may have anaesthesia in the area.

Paroxysmal Glossopharyngeal Neuralgia: This condition occurs very much less commonly than paroxysmal trigeminal neuralgia and may be associated with vagal neuralgia.

Aetiology

Even less is known about the aetiology of the condition than of paroxysmal trigeminal neuralgia.

Clinical features

Paroxysmal glossopharyngeal neuralgia may be divided into:
  a. Otic—where the pain is mainly related to the ear.
  b. Pharyngeal—with the pain at the angle of the jaw in the throat or upper part of the neck. The paroxysmal feature is not so striking as in paroxysmal trigeminal neuralgia, but the pain may be triggered by swallowing, talking or even movement of the tongue. Vagal features have been described, including nausea, sometimes vomiting and even bradycardia occurring in paroxysms.

Differential diagnosis

The otic type must be differentiated from pain due to lesions of the ear and the pharyngeal type from other lesions of the oropharynx. A condition called 'stylalgia' has been described where the pain is thought to be due to an elongated styloid process with calcification of the stylopharyngeal ligament. Pain is experienced on movement of the head. The elongated styloid process can be seen on X-ray.

Treatment

Carbamazepine may be effective, and is given in the same dose as for paroxysmal trigeminal neuralgia. If this is not effective a surgical approach is needed, with section of nerve or tract by the neurosurgeon.

Periodic Migrainous Neuralgia

Periodic migrainous neuralgia is a facial pain of vascular origin which is best regarded as a form of migraine, the uniting feature of all the various migrainous syndromes being vascular constriction and dilatation. This is due to a biochemical abnormality, the exact nature of which is not known. Migrainous headaches are due to involvement of the internal carotid artery. It would appear that basilar migraine is due to involvement of the basilar artery and ophthalmoplegic migraine to involvement of the ophthalmic artery. Periodic migrainous neuralgia appears to be an involvement of the external carotid artery, more specifically the maxillary division. All these conditions have features common to migraine but are recognized by the associated symptoms and signs which vary according to the vessel involved.

There are a large number of conditions which have been described over the years, all of which are not regarded as bascially periodic migrainous neuralgia. Much time in learning the subject can be saved by recognizing the synonyms. Horton's headache or syndrome, Slüder's neuralgia or syndrome, histamine encephalgia or headache, cluster headache, hemifacial migrainous neuralgia, sphenopalatine syndrome, Harris' headache or neuralgia, cilary ganglion syndrome and 'alarm clock headache' are all the same condition.

Aetiology

Many of the aetiological features of migraine are seen in the patient with periodic migrainous neuralgia, the patient often giving a history of migraine or cyclical vomiting as a child. Such patients often have a conscientious, perfectionist type of personality. Intellectually they have difficulty in keeping up with the standard they set themselves. Although migraine is more common in women, for some unknown reason periodic migrainous neuralgia is far more common in men, many of the patients being students. A wide age group is affected, usually starting in the second decade and may persist into the fifth and rarely sixth decades. The mechanism of migraine, consisting of arteriospasm followed by dilatation, has been confirmed by angiograph. Temporal artery biopsies have shown that the wall of the artery becomes thickened, which impairs the blood supply, followed by a reflex dilatation. A number of chemical substances have been investigated as causative agents by their local action on the vessels concerned. Among these are various kinins, e.g. 'neurokinin' and 5-hydroxytryptamine (serotonin).

In the case of periodic migrainous neuralgia, it has been suggested that the vessel involved is that supplying the sphenopalatine ganglion.

Clinical features

The pain starts suddenly, being described as extremely severe with a throbbing, burning or boring nature. Generally the pain starts around one eye and spreads to involve the whole of that side of the face, extending on occasions into the temporal region. When the pain starts the patient is often nauseated but rarely vomits. In most cases the pain is confined to one side of the face but in some subsequent attacks may occur on the other side of the face. Attacks generally occur once in 24 hours, commonly at night, hence the name 'alarm clock headache' when it will wake the patient at the same time for several nights. The pain lasts about an hour, though some attacks last longer. More than one attack per day is not rare and the attacks can become so close that they are almost continuous. Attacks occur in bouts which last from a few days to a few months. The condition occurs at regular intervals at first, but later becomes irregular and finally stops, only to resume a few months later. There may be remissions of several years.

Associated phenomena: Along with the facial pain there are a number of associated phenomena. The side of the face affected feels hot and may even sweat. Unilateral epiphora and a sensation of nasal blockage may occur with rhinorrhoea. There may even be unilateral photophobia. If the patient sees his face in a mirror at the time of the attack he will notice that there is unilateral conjunctivitis, with erythema of the affected side of the face. During the attack the face may be tender to pressure.

Not all the associated phenomena occur in every case and diagnosis may have to be made on the pain with only one or two associated phenomena.

Differential diagnosis

In a case with a classical history there is very little else that this collection of features could suggest. The difficulty comes when features are missing or the patient gives a poor history. X-rays of the maxillary sinus should be taken to exclude sinusitis and it is generally wise to have full mouth dental films taken in all but the most classical cases, so that a dental cause can be excluded. Two serious conditions must always be borne in mind: retrobulbar neuritis and cranial arteritis. In retrobulbar neuritis the pain is continuous, always occurring around the eye with tenderness of the globe. The patient may even vomit. Eventually a scotoma (an area of blindness) develops in the affected eye. In cranial arteritis there is extreme tenderness over the affected artery. The condition may spread to involve the central artery of the retina with resulting blindness. This is a condition of elderly people where periodic migrainous neuralgia is in the middle age group. Both retrobulbar neuritis and cranial arteritis give a high ESR, usually above 60 mm in the first hour. ACTH or prednisone should be given if either of these conditions is suspected.

Acute glaucoma may present with severe pain in and around the eye, which may be intermittent at first. Like periodic migrainous neuralgia, the pain may be very severe and may even cause vomiting, which is rare in periodic migrainous neuralgia. Vision is reduced and this reduction may be preceded by the perception of halos and lights. The eye itself is congested and has a dusky appearance. Usually the pupil is dilated and will not respond to light. On palpation the globe of the eye is either very painful or hard.

If there is any doubt about the eye in a patient with suspected periodic migrainous neuralgia, the patient should be given 1 per cent eserine eye drops and analgesics and arrangements should be made for him to see an ophthalmologist as soon as possible.

Treatment

It is naïve to think that any migrainous condition will respond to one specific remedy in all patients. A number of different regimes may need to be given a reasonable therapeutic trial before a treatment is found which will suit the patient.

Ergot derivatives: There are many proprietary preparations commonly used in migraine which are often effective in periodic migrainous neuralgia. Most contain ergotamine 1–2 mg, caffeine 100 mg and some have added antiemetic, anticholinergic or analgesic drugs. The caffeine is almost traditional as an adjunct, but it has been suggested recently that it can potentiate pain. Subcutaneous ergotamine tartrate 0·5 mg, suppositories and inhalations of a solution (Medihaler-Ergotamine) have also been tried and all have their exponents. In common they share the dangers of the ergot derivatives, causing vascular spasm, and are contraindicated in cases of peripheral vascular disease, hypertension or myocardial insufficiency. It would be unwise to give these during pregnancy. There is a danger in all cases of the patient taking an overdose, causing angina or peripheral paraesthesia of the limbs due to vascular spasm.

Methysergide (Deseril): This drug is an antagonist of 5-hydroxytryptamine. A dose of 1 mg tds could be doubled with good prophylactic effect. It has many of the same side effects as the ergot derivatives and is contraindicated in the same cases. Prolonged administration has led to retroperitoneal fibrosis, which may cause a silent hydronephrosis.

Clonidine 0·025 mg tds is safer and as effective.

Sedatives and tranquillizers: These can also be used prophylactically. Chlordiazepoxide may be given by day and a barbiturate by night.

Antihistamines: These seem to have some place, especially those which also have a hypnotic action, e.g. promethazine hydrochloride (Phenergan) 50 mg nocte.

Antidepressants: Amitriptyline 75 mg nocte may be useful.

Atypical Facial Pain

Definition

A poorly-localized, vague but occasionally dramatic facial pain of functional origin. It may represent an important aspect of depression.

Introduction

There is much confusion in the early literature on atypical facial pain. Many efforts have been made to explain it on an organic basis, e.g. temporomandibular joint dysfunction and vasomotor phenomena. Added to this, some cases described as atypical facial pain can now quite clearly be seen as periodic migrainous neuralgia. Other clinicians have either denied the existence of the disease or claimed it as a variant of paroxysmal trigeminal neuralgia.

Aetiology

This is complex and our knowledge on the subject is still incomplete. There are many functional diseases which can present as pain with the face forming a focus. In no way is this surprising, as the face is an extremely important part of personal anatomy and is the only part of the body which can portray the character of the person. Thus, in simple terms, if a person has 'psychological pain' it is not surprising if this pain is located in the face. An important step in understanding this condition came when it was realized that there were many manifestations of endogenous depression and pain was an important factor. The following have been cited as functional causes of atypical facial pain.

Endogenous depression: Atypical facial pain may be seen in a classical endogenous depression when the patient may appear depressed, wake early in the morning or be unable to sleep and lose the appetite for food and sex. Such patients may be self-critical with feelings of self-reproach which may even proceed to delusions of punishment. Suicidal ideas are common in this group of patients.

Atypical depression: Here many of the classical features of endogenous depression are obscured and the dominant features are those of fatigue, irritability and lethargy. Atypical facial pain is perhaps more commonly found in this group of patients.

Anxiety neurosis (or anxiety state): The patient may be aware of the psychological tension that is developing within him; this may precipitate a wide spectrum of physical symptoms, of which facial pain is one. This is sometimes known as an 'organ neurosis' and is commonly seen before an important event in a person's life, e.g. 'butterflies in the stomach'. In atypical facial pain the organ may be the face, as part of a chronic anxiety state.

Obsessional neurosis: Here thoughts and feelings cannot be removed from the mind. Many patients with atypical facial pain have features of an obsessional personality. These patients are more preoccupied with symptoms than are the usual run of people. A minor dental symptom may be exaggerated out of all proportion or recognition.

Hysteria: This is a very rare cause of atypical facial pain: the patient's symptoms must be initiated and potentiated for the gain which he obtains from them. Occasionally such patients have a doting relative who is perhaps more concerned about the pain than is the patient himself, and will wait on the patient hand and foot, especially when the pain is present. For some reason, most hysterical features involve other parts of the body rather than the face, e.g. the heart.

The above account is an oversimplification of a number of complex components which may be mixed in a most confusing manner.

Clinical features

Over 70 per cent of cases of atypical facial pain occur in women of all ages, but there are two peaks, one around 20 and the other at the menopause. Many of the patients have had their symptoms for many years, visiting many medical specialists in an attempt to gain relief. Nearly all these patients have had a considerable amount of dental treatment, generally to little avail.

The facial pain is usually unilateral, but it can be bilateral and although more common in the maxilla, it may involve any part of the facial complex. It is well worth mapping out the area where the pain occurs. Quite often there are anatomical incongruities with bizarre distributions, often crossing the midline in a tell-tale way.

Many different types of pain are described, but usually it is a severe dull ache which becomes worse at times. Some patients even have two types of pain, one dull and the other severe. On occasions the pain may be replaced by altered sensations such as formication (sensation of insects crawling under the skin), burning sensation or paraesthesia. In the majority of cases the pain is intermittent, but in a surprising number the pain may be continuous over years. Most patients seem to sleep well in spite of the pain, but some give dramatic histories of how they have been unable to sleep for years because of the pain.

Analgesics do very little to relieve the pain, nor can the patient find any relief, although a few obsessional patients have a bizarre ritual which they claim gives them relief. Pain is quite commonly precipitated by anxiety and worry.

Although physical findings are essentially negative, it is quite common to discover a number of minor dental faults.

Diagnosis

A careful history is the key to the diagnosis. The clinician must be prepared to sit down in a quiet room for an hour without a large audience, if he is to obtain a useful history from these patients. Once the patient sees that the investigator is sympathetic to his complaints and is prepared to follow up each point, then more relevant information will follow. As much information as possible must be gained about the patient's psychiatric history. A useful lead in this direction is to ask the patient if he suffers from his nerves. Once the ice has been broken on this subject, the information will flow. The way in which the patient gives the information may be very instructive. Depressed patients may appear to have given up hope, but may, if suffering from an atypical depression, show irritability and annoyance. The obsessional patient will tend to give every detail of the history with precision, even to the point of having dates recorded. The hysterical patient will give a dramatic history with frequent use of superlatives to describe the pain. In cases where there is an anxiety component, stress and anxiety often make the pain worse.

Every effort must be made to exclude all organic lesions. Minor dental and periodontal pathology should be treated first. Features of temporomandibular joint dysfunction should be sought specifically. Cervical spondylitis must be borne in mind and, where indicated, X-ray of the cervical spine should be requested. No patient should proceed to any treatment without having full X-rays of the teeth so that all the apices can be seen and also X-rays of the maxillary sinuses. It would be tragic to misdiagnose a nasopharyngeal carcinoma as atypical facial pain.

A full physical examination will often prove helpful in difficult cases and perhaps ought to form part of the routine examination of these patients. It may be that only during the actual examination will the patient admit to pain in other regions of the body. Once the investigator has taken an interest in the whole patient, other information which helps considerably may be released.

It is never satisfactory to make a diagnosis of atypical facial pain on negative features only. Ideally, all patients should be seen by a psychiatrist at some stage, but many patients still have resistance to this type of consultation.

Course and prognosis

Where there is an obsessional or an hysterical component the prognosis is poor. Many of the other patients will make an initial improvement only to relapse, but perhaps next time with abdominal pain or backache. There is a great danger that when a diagnosis of atypical facial pain has been made the patient's future complaints will be attributed to functional causes. Neurosis and psychosis do not confer immunity to dental caries, periodontal or any other disease.

Treatment

To obtain the best results, the aetiology must be determined and treatment undertaken in conjunction with the psychiatrist.

In cases where there is an anxiety component, minor tranquillizers are the drugs of choice. Chlordiazepoxide (Librium) 10 mg bd or tds (the dose can safely be doubled) is an extremely safe drug, contraindicated only in patients with renal or hepatic failure and in the very old. Diazepam (Valium) 5 mg bd or tds (again, doses can safely be doubled) may also be employed, the contraindications being as above, with the addition that it should not be given to patients with a history of glaucoma.

Where there is a history of anergic endogenous depression, imipramine 25–50 mg tds is given until the depression starts to lift, followed by 25 mg bd, tailing off at three months, is often effective. Quite often depressed patients have anxiety features and amitriptyline and its derivatives are best in this group of patients; alternatively, prothiaden in the same dosage (75–150 mg nocte) is less sedating.

Patients with atypical depression do not respond so well to the tricyclic antidepressants and it may be necessary to give them monoamine oxidase inhibitors with all their inherent dangers. In skilled hands, coupled with warning the patient about the dangers, these drugs can be made relatively safe. Protriptyline (Concordin) 5–10 mg tds may be successful where other tricyclic antidepressants fail. Only occasionally is it necessary to proceed to ECT in resistance cases.

Constant review of patients is a difficult problem. In some patients a periodic watch is needed for changing features with possible organic causes, but on the other hand there is a feeling that this helps to potentiate the patient's symptoms. There is much to be said for treating what can be treated and then discharging the patient when he is symptom-free.

Bibliography

Bella J. I. and Walton J. N. (1964) Periodic migranous neuralgia. *Br. Med. J.* **1**, 219.

Blom S. (1962) Trigeminal neuralgia: its treatment with a new anticonvulsant drug (G-32883). *Lancet* **1**, 839.

Bohm E. and Strang R. R. (1962) Glossopharyngeal neuralgia. *Brain* **85**, 371.

Burke W. J. G. and Selby G. (1965) Trigeminal neuralgia, a therapeutic trial with Tegretol. *Proc. Aust. Assoc. Neurol.* **3**, 89.

Chawla J. C. and Falconer W. A. (1967) Glossopharyngeal and vagal neuralgia. *Br. Med. J.* **2**, 529.

Dimsdale H. (1967) Migraine. *Practitioner* **198**, 490.

Engel S. L. (1951) Primary atypical facial neuralgias. An hysterical conversion symptom. *Psychosom. Med.* **13**, 375.

Engel S. L. (1959) Psychogenic pain and the pain-prone patient. *Am. J. Med.* **26**, 899.

Gayford J. J. (1969) Atypical facial pain. *Practitioner* **202**, 657.

Graham J. G. (1967) Trigeminal neuralgia. *Practitioner* **198**, 497.

Harris W. (1940) An analysis of 1433 cases of paroxysmal trigeminal neuralgia, and end result of Gausserian alcohol injection. *Brain* **63**, 209.

Lascelles R. G. (1966) Atypical facial pain. *Br. J. Psychiat.* **112,** 651.
Merskey H. and Spear F. G. (1967) *Pain: Psychological and Psychiatric Aspects.* London, Ballière, Tindall and Cox.
Parkes J. D. (1975) Relief of pain: headache, facial neuralgia, migraine and phantom limb. *Br. Med. J.* **2,** 90.
Spillane J. D. (1964) Treatment of trigeminal neuralgia: preliminary experiences with Tegretol. *Practitioner* **192,** 71.

Chapter 18

Facial Pain. IV. Neurological Diseases Affecting the Trigeminal Nerve

In this chapter the diseases associated with symptoms and signs of trigeminal nerve involvement are described. The symptoms are pain and anaesthesia in the distribution of the nerve and the objective evidence of demonstrable sensory deficit in the trigeminal area and possible motor weakness of the supplied muscles (masticatory, mylohyoid and anterior belly of digastric).

Lesions affecting the *facial nerve* and those principally affecting facial muscles—myasthenia, myopathies and motor neurone disease—are considered in Chapter 19.

The contents of this chapter will be subdivided into consideration of the affections of the mandibular division, the maxillary division outside the skull, and intracranial lesions.

The Mandibular Division

This section is an account of the peripheral disorders affecting essentially the inferior dental nerve, so giving rise to anaesthesia of the lower lip. There will also be passing consideration given to the involvement of the lingual and auriculotemporal nerves.

The extracranial causes of anaesthesia of the lower lip are most readily considered by following the nerve supply of the lower lip from the mental foramen to the skull, with three anatomical subdivisions, namely:

a. The mental nerve.
b. The inferior dental nerve within the mandible.
c. The inferior dental nerve and mandibular trunk from the mandibular foramen to the skull base (foramen ovale).

The mental nerve

The mental nerve is commonly damaged in operations in the lower premolar region. If the nerve is stretched or compressed, recovery is rapid within a few days but actual severance of the nerve is associated with more profound and prolonged anaesthesia and recovery is heralded by hyperaesthesia and paraesthesia.

Periapical abscesses of the lower premolars may involve the mental nerve with anaesthesia of the lower lip and appropriate treatment leads to rapid remission. Such a diagnosis must not be made lightly and careful follow up is required to ensure that osteomyelitis is not overlooked.

In such involvement of the mental nerve the incisive branch is spared and so the gingiva of the incisor region retains its normal sensibility.

The inferior dental nerve within the mandible

The inferior dental nerve within the mandible may be damaged in association with a fracture of the body of the mandible, but the obvious features of the associated injury point to the correct diagnosis. Trauma to the inferior dental nerve also occurs as a result of removal of impacted wisdom teeth and in other operations affecting the mandible. That nerve damage is likely to occur is clearly evidence in the pre-operative radiograph and the patient should be forewarned of its occurrence as this considerably reduces the subjective disturbance associated with this symptom. In the majority of cases the inferior dental nerve is simply 'tweaked' and the resultant neuropraxia remits within a fortnight. Neurotmesis follows extraction of a tooth in which there is an intimate relationship between the nerve and the root of the tooth. In such cases the mental anaesthesia is total and may be associated with painful paraesthesia; recovery takes up to six months and may never be complete. Exceptionally, severe paraesthesia plagues the patient for many years. Removal of wisdom teeth may also be associated with neuropraxia of the lingual nerve which remits in a few days and exceptionally the nerve is severed, which leads to prolonged, often permanent, anaesthesia of the ipsilateral half of the tongue. This is a formidable sensory deficit for any patient to bear and is always avoidable. Conversely, permanent mental anaesthesia from such cause is not always avoidable but leads to little, if any, distress to the patient. A cardinal sign of *osteomyelitis* of the mandible is anaesthesia of the same half of the lower lip which is not seen with simple periapical suppuration or dry socket. There are always other features such as pain, swelling, discharging sinuses and, after the first fortnight, radiographic evidence of bone destruction.

Malignant tumours invading the mandible lead to early anaesthesia of the lip, although this symptom may be associated with severe radiating pain which precedes the anaesthesia. There may be swelling of the mandible in the affected area but there is *always* evidence of central bone destruction on the radiograph. Such a clinical picture may be due to primary central malignancy such as carcinoma arising in a dental cyst, or an adenocarcinoma or an osteosarcoma, but is more commonly due to metastases and may be due to myelomatous or leukaemic deposits. Exceptionally, the lesion is benign—either an acutely infected dental cyst or benign neural sheath tumours of the inferior dental nerve.

The inferior dental nerve (or mandibular trunk) from the mandible to the skull base

The inferior dental nerve (or mandibular trunk) from the mandible to the skull base is at risk during inferior dental nerve block injection. Damage of this nerve (or the lingual) may be produced by the needle or by any fluid carried in the needle and deposited around the nerves. The patient complains of persistent anaesthesia, usually of a small area on the lip. In such a case there is no trismus or pain; and gradual recovery over a few months is usual. The injection may, however, also be complicated by haematoma formation or infection and then the persistent anaesthesia is associated with trismus and pain at the injection site. This remits over the succeeding week or two with the help of antibiotics in infective cases.

The mandibular division of the trigeminal may be involved by a *carcinoma* invading the lateral wall of the nasopharynx which produces *Trotter's syndrome*. The carcinoma occludes the Eustachian tube to cause deafness and invades the levator palati, which leads to elevation but immobility of the soft palate. The mandibular division is infiltrated, thereby causing neuralgic pain radiating along the course of the inferior dental, lingual and auriculotemporal nerves associated with anaesthesia of the lower lip and tongue. The patient is usually an elderly man and craggy upper deep cervical lymphadenopathy may be noted. On occasion, the tumour invades superiorly rather than laterally to involve the maxillary division rather than the mandibular. Diagnosis is effected by endoscopy and biopsy under general anaesthesia.

The Maxillary Division

The maxillary division may be involved in Trotter's syndrome as noted above but the two common causes of anaesthesia of the cheek are due to involvement of the infra-orbital nerve in either maxillary fractures or carcinoma of the maxillary antrum. Carcinoma of the antrum may also be associated with pain in the distribution of the infra-orbital nerve or its posterior, middle or anterior dental branches. Diagnosis is obvious in either case from the associated clinical features.

Intracranial Lesions

Intracranial lesions producing symptoms and signs attributable to involvement of the trigeminal nerve and presenting to the dental surgeon are quite exceptional, and correspondingly the emphasis will be on the suspicious features which should lead to full neurological investigation. They will be considered under the following headings:

1. Space-occupying lesions.
2. Disseminated (multiple) sclerosis.
3. Cerebrovascular diseases.
4. Syringobulbia.
5. Syphilis, tabes dorsalis.
6. Benign trigeminal neuropathy.
7. Stilbamidine neuropathy.
8. Hysteria.

1. *Space-occupying lesions*

The commonest tumour affecting the trigeminal nerve, the acoustic neuroma, occupies the cerebellopontine angle and will be described as a prototype although a similar clinical picture will be produced by meningiomas, angiomas, aneurysms or 'cholesteatomas'.

As a first symptom, deafness is not uncommon but may pass unnoticed by the patient and then progressive sensory loss in the face antedates other symptoms. Pain may occur in the distribution of the trigeminal nerve but is unusual; when present it is normally persistent but occasionally may simulate trigeminal neuralgia. Tinnitus may occur.

Symptoms of labyrinthine disturbance such as vertigo and unsteadiness may occur, similarly facial weakness which is progressive. Involvement of the adjacent brain stem leads to contralateral upper motor neurone damage evidenced in spastic weakness of the leg and arm. Early evidence of raised intracranial pressure such as headache and papilloedema due to disturbance of the ventricular system with obstructive hydrocephalus may occur. These symptoms are more commonly late features.

Examination reveals that the trigeminal deficit is sensory and involves pain sensation to a greater extent than light touch. The corneal reflex is characteristically absent. A unilateral perceptive deafness is almost essential to the diagnosis and there is also labyrinthine paresis. This is associated with nystagmus towards the affected side. Facial nerve involvement evidenced by weakness of facial muscles may be present. If the long tracts are involved there is spastic weakness of the opposite leg with an extensor (Babinski) plantar response.

The cardinal signs may, therefore, be summarized as:

a. Hypoaesthesia within the trigeminal area.
b. Absent corneal reflex.
c. Perceptive deafness.
d. Nystagmus.
e. Facial weakness.
f. Contralateral *extensor* plantar response.

Lesions of the middle cranial fossa affecting the trigeminal ganglion and trunks may be meningiomas, angiomas, aneurysms or metastatic deposits. Symptomatically these differ from posterior fossa lesions in that both sensory and motor functions of the trigeminal nerve are affected. The sensory deficit demonstrably affects pain and light touch equally and there is atrophy of the muscles of mastication on the affected side with failure to contract on clenching the teeth. Other cranial nerves involved may be those to the extra-ocular muscles, particularly the abducent, producing a lateral rectus palsy.

The cardinal features are thus:

a. Hypoaesthesia (trigeminal area).
b. Weakness of muscles of mastication.
c. Lateral rectus palsy.

In either case with suggestive features, the opinion of a neurologist must be sought and after appropriate investigation, treatment is neurosurgical.

2. *Disseminated (multiple) sclerosis*

The central connections of the trigeminal nerve may be involved in a plaque of demyelination to cause an area of numbness on the face or weakness of the muscles of mastication. On occasion the disease produces a syndrome indistinguishable from trigeminal neuralgia in young subjects. Usually there are other lesions characteristically distinct in place and time which allow diagnosis, but if a unilateral sensory loss of the face is the first and only sign the diagnosis only becomes apparent with the passage of time.

3. *Cerebrovascular diseases*

Affecting the brain stem may produce striking syndromes expressed mainly in the face, principally occlusion of the posterior inferior cerebellar artery (due to embolism or thrombosis), which leads to a clinical picture called Wallenberg's syndrome. There is sudden or rapidly progressive evidence of involvement of the V descending nucleus, vagus and the ipsilateral sympathetic system and cerebellum. Of the tracts running through the medulla the spinothalamic tract is that principally involved. The symptoms are of unilateral loss of pain and temperature sensation on the face with the same symptom on the opposite half of the body due to involvement of the crossed spinothalamic tract. The affected side of the face also exhibits a Horner's syndrome (sympathetic palsy) and paralysis of the soft palate. Signs of cerebellar disturbance are also demonstrable on the same side of the body.

Involvement of the anterior inferior cerebellar artery produces ipsilateral sensory loss due to nuclear ischaemia with destruction of the nuclei of the facial and auditory nerves also, leading to facial palsy and deafness with labyrinthine disturbance (nausea, vertigo and nystagmus). To this is added ipsilateral cerebellar disturbance and Horner's syndrome and involvement of the spinothalamic tract as in Wallenberg's syndrome.

4. *Syringobulbia*

In this disease (the 'brain stem analogue of syringomyelia) there is early involvement of the descending fibres from the trigeminal nerve of each side to its spinal nucleus. This leads to gradually extending loss of sensibility to pain and temperature involving the ophthalmic division to a greater extent but spreading from the periphery of the whole face to converge upon the nose. In addition there is a lower motor neurone palsy affecting the vagus, hypoglossal and accessory nerves, manifested principally in the motor supply to the larynx and pharynx. With progression there is an upper motor neurone lesion affecting the lower and upper limbs manifested in spastic weakness; even in the earliest cases the plantar responses may be extensor. Thus all the signs are bilateral but may be asymmetrical at first.

5. *Syphilis*

In meningiovascular syphilis there may be an involvement of the trigeminal ganglion as in middle cranial fossa tumours, but nerves supplying the extra-ocular muscles are extensively involved.

In the *tabes dorsalis* the characteristic features in the head and neck are a patch of sensory loss to pain extending from the nose slightly over the adjacent cheeks, and Argyll–Robertson pupils, which are small and irregular, reacting sluggishly, if at all, to light but normally to accommodation. Exceptionally the lightning pains of tabes may be manifested in the distribution of the trigeminal nerve and may be mistaken for trigeminal neuralgia. Such a mistake is not perpetuated beyond the subsequent neurological examination which, as mentioned elsewhere, is entirely negative in idiopathic trigeminal neuralgia.

In *general paralysis of the insane* there are dysarthria and coarse antero-posterior tremor of the tongue.

Diagnosis in all such cases is affected by serological tests of blood and cerebrospinal fluid. The basis of treatment is 28 daily injections of 600 000 units of procaine penicillin.

6. *Benign sensory trigeminal neuropathy*

This disorder of unknown aetiology, although rare, is nethertheless one of the commonest central afflictions of the trigeminal nerve presenting to the dental surgeon. Although classed as 'central', the site of the lesion and its cause are quite unknown except that in chronic cases explored by Hughes, he found the sensory root of the trigeminal ganglion reduced to a few fibres which were degenerate and some chronic inflammatory cells.

It is probable that there are included several distinct clinico-pathological entities that (in common with many such problems in medicine) will only be unravelled by a prospective cooperative international study over a period of at least ten years.

Clinical features: The symptom complex which occurs at any age is characterized by a fairly abrupt onset with pain in the face, either maxilla or mandible, which radiates within the area of distribution of the affected division, and teeth are frequently removed at this stage without relief. Within a few days there is noted an area of anaesthesia, often in the infra-orbital or mental nerve area, and this gradually extends and there may be associated paraesthesia. Exceptionally the anaesthesia extends to involve the whole trigeminal nerve on one side, but usually is limited to one division and even then is rarely complete.

Examination confirms that the sensory loss in the trigeminal area is the only neurological abnormality. Rarely there may be some weakness of the ipsilateral muscles of mastication which may, however, be an expression of sensory (proprioceptive) deficit.

Diagnosis can only be confidently made with a most careful neurological examination and follow up is essential.

In the majority of cases the symptoms and signs persist for a few weeks and then slowly regress over two to four months. In a few cases, however, especially in those with a gradual onset, there may be permanent anaesthesia with or without neuralgic pains and paraesthesia for many years. In view of this variable outlook the initial prognosis in any case should be guarded.

7. *Stilbamidine neuropathy*

Stilbamidine is a diamidine drug (analagous to pentamidine) which is effective in trypanosomiasis, leishmaniasis and as an antifungal agent in blastomycosis. In addition to being potent releasers of tissue histamine, the drugs are neurotoxic. Hydroxystilbamidine has the added distinction of causing a bilateral sensory trigeminal neuropathy in well over 50 per cent of cases. This is characterized by anaesthesia and paraesthesia and neuralgic pains and appears to be permanent in most cases. Similar sensory neuropathy affecting other parts of the body may be noted.

8. *Hysteria*

In this disorder any neurological symptom may be present including anaesthesia of the face. Characteristically the anaesthesia is bilateral and does not quite fit the distribution of the trigeminal nerve. There may also be other bizarre neurological features, but on occasion the diagnosis may be very difficult to establish (in a hysterical neurologist it would be impossible). Treatment ideally is psychological, but most of the patients find this unacceptable. The part played by psychological disturbances in the aetiology of facial pain (atypical facial pain) is considered in the next chapter.

Bibliography

Blau J. N., Harris M. and Kennett S. (1969) Trigeminal sensory neuropathy. *N. Engl. J. Med.* **281,** 873.

Brain W. R. (1962) *Diseases of the Nervous System.* London, Oxford University Press.

Goldstein N. P., Gibilisco J. A. and Rushton J. G. (1963) Trigeminal neuropathy and neuritis. *JAMA* **184,** 458.

Harris M. (1967) Disturbances of facial sensation. *Oral Surg.* **24,** 335.

Hughes B. (1958) Chronic benign trigeminal paresis. *Proc. R. Soc. Med.* **51,** 529.

Jefferson G. (1953) The differential diagnosis of lesions of the posterior fossa. *Proc. R. Soc. Med.* **46,** 719.

Seward M. (1962) Anaesthesia of the lower lip. *Br. Dent. J.* **113,** 423.

Chapter 19

Facial Neuropathy

Anatomy (*Fig.* 6)

Although on pure anatomical grounds there is good foundation for dividing the facial nerve into the facial nerve proper and the nervus intermedius, clinically it is more convenient to divide the nerve into four parts as follows:

Motor   1. The facial nerve proper.

            2. The secreto motor part of the facial nerve.

Sensory   3. The nervus intermedius part of the facial nerve associated with taste.

            4. Sensory component.

1. *The facial nerve proper*

This is the part of the facial nerve which innervates the musculature of the face including the orbicularis oculi, orbicularis oris and the buccinator muscles. It also innervates the muscles of the scalp and auricle. The platysma, stapedius and stylohyoid muscles are, with the posterior belly of the digastric, in a like manner innervated by the facial nerve.

Deep in the pons is the facial nucleus, which receives fibres from the contralateral corticonuclear (corticopontine) tract. As the upper part of the face is bilaterally innervated the facial nucleus must also receive some fibres from the ipsilateral corticonuclear tract. In their passage from the appropriate motor area of the cerebral cortex, corticonuclear fibres have to pass through the internal capsule with many other fibres, all of which are damaged by haemorrhage in this region.

The innervation of emotional expression is still imperfectly understood but there appears to be essential connection with the frontal and temporal regions of the brain. Probably the corpus striatum plays a part, as is shown in Parkinsonism.

Leaving the pons at the cerebellopontine angle, the facial nerve enters the internal auditory canal with the eighth cranial nerve. It passes into the

234

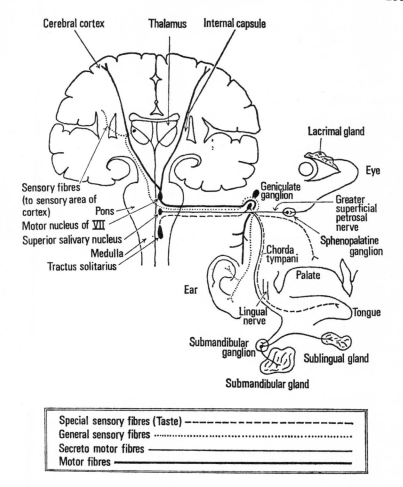

Fig. 6. Pathways of the facial nerve.

petrous part of the temporal bone in the facial or fallopian canal. Still inside the bone, the nerve turns at right angles to its original course; as it turns there is an enlargement of the nerve formed by the geniculate ganglion. Still in its bony canal, the nerve passes backwards and downwards along the medial wall of the tympanic antrum giving a branch to the stapedius muscle and leaving the skull through the stylomastoid foramen, posterior to the styloid process. Finally the nerve enters the parotid gland where it divides into its terminal branches to supply muscles of the face.

2. *The secretomotor part of the facial nerve*

Fibres arising in the superior salivary nucleus of the pons leave the brain with the facial nerve, but in a separate nerve termed the nervus intermedius. This joins the facial nerve at the geniculate ganglion, but the secretomotor fibres do not relay in the ganglion; instead they pass straight into the greater superficial petrosal nerve. Thus secretomotor fibres traverse the petrous temporal bone to reach the sphenopalatine ganglion. In this ganglion the nerve does synapse with its terminal branches innervating the lacrimal gland, glands in the nose and even the palate.

Not all secretomotor fibres leave the facial nerve at the geniculate ganglion; some travel further in the nerve to leave via the chorda tympani where they eventually join the lingual nerve. From the lingual nerve, fibres pass to the submandibular ganglion where they relay before innervating the submandibular and sublingual salivary glands.

This part of the facial nerve forms part of the parasympathetic nervous system and transmission along these nerves will be affected by drugs which have an action on autonomic nervous conduction (*see* Chapter 13).

3. *The part of the facial nerve associatad with taste*

Taste buds in the anterior two-thirds of the tongue have efferent fibres which pass in the lingual nerve to join the chorda tympani and progress to the geniculate ganglion. Other taste buds in the palate transmit their impulses via the palatine nerves to the sphenopalatine ganglion and greater superficial petrosal nerve to reach the geniculate ganglion. All taste nerves relay in the geniculate ganglion before passing centrally via the facial nerve to the tractus solitarius in the medulla oblongata. Finally, efferent fibres pass to the thalamus of the contralateral side and relay to the postcentral gyrus. Taste must be regarded as the special sensory component of the facial nerve.

4. *The sensory component of the facial nerve*

On clinical grounds, as suggested by the Ramsay-Hunt syndrome, there is a pure sensory component of the facial nerve, which originates from the tympanic membrane, external auditory meatus and part of the pinna of the ear. There are probably a number of sensory communications between the terminal branches of the facial and trigeminal nerve. Sensory fibres probably relay in the geniculate ganglion as they pass centrally to the contralateral higher centres of the brain.

Clinical Examination of the Facial Nerve and Musculature

The clinical examination starts the moment the patient or the clinician enters the room. Observations made while the patient is talking or otherwise occupied can be very helpful.

Inspection

The symmetry of the face is best seen as the patient is talking. It may be obvious that wrinkles have been lost on one-half of the forehead or that the patient is not blinking. Both these features are more commonly seen when the lesion is in the pons or lower as the upper part of the face is bilaterally innervated. Movement of the mouth as the patient speaks is important, especially when they allow themselves the luxury of some emotional expression. The twitch or tremor of uncontrolled emotional expression must be further investigated. The same applies to lack of emotional expression with voluntary motor function retained. Patients with a long-standing lower motor neurone facial palsy may have developed a contraction which can give the paralysed side of the face the appearance of a smile. At a cursory glance it would be easy to mistake the side of the palsy unless the movement of the face is carefully watched. The absence of the nasolabial fold is very obvious in patients with normally strong facial features.

Examination of motor function

Basically the facial musculature can be divided into two components, examined separately.

a. *Upper part* (round the eyes and forehead): If the patient is asked to close his eyes the palsy may become obvious, with the affected eyelids failing to close and the globe turning up so that only the white of the eye is showing. Weakness of orbicularis muscles with sufficient strength to close the eyes can be compared with the normal side by asking the patient to close his eyes tight and observing the degree of force required

238 CLINICAL ORAL MEDICINE

to part the eyelids. If the patient is asked to wrinkle his forehead weakness can be detected by the difference between the two sides. The significance of the upper part of the face being affected has already been stressed.

b. Lower part (round the mouth): This is best examined by asking the patient to smile, bare his teeth or to purse his lips. Any effort to blow out the cheeks will be spoiled by the lack of lip seal and an accompanying sound of escaping air.

c. Testing corneal reflex: This depends on the integrity of the trigeminal and facial nerve, either of which being defective will give a negative response.

d. Testing taste: In the main this is a most unsatisfactory procedure. Four distinctive-tasting substances are required, preferably without smell. A sweet solution, a salt solution, an acid solution such as vinegar and solution of peppermint, are the traditional test materials even though the latter has a smell. The patient is asked to protrude his tongue and the anterior two-thirds is touched with a pledget of cotton wool moistened with test substance. Each test must be made laterally and usually the patient has to draw his tongue back in his mouth before being able to make a comment. As can be seen, this method of testing is open to great error, and the significance of unilateral loss of taste associated with facial palsy is not as great as was once considered, but indicates that the facial nerve is involved above the chorda tympani.

e. Hearing: Hyperacusis may be caused by paralysis of the stapedius muscle. Again this may be difficult to assess. The only significance is again that the level of the lesion is placed above the branching of the nerve to stapedius.

f. Lacrimation: This is tested by hooking a 3 mm wide strip of litmus paper in the lower conjunctival fornix. The strip should dampen to at least 15 mm in one minute if tear production is normal. The contralateral eye serves as a control (Schirmer's test).

Secretion is diminished in lesions of the facial nerve involving the geniculate ganglion or in the internal auditory meatus.

Causes of Facial Palsy

Supranuclear (upper motor neurone) lesions give rise to facial palsy which involves only the lower two-thirds of the face. Nuclear and infranuclear (lower motor neurone) lesions give a palsy which affects both the upper and lower parts of the face. Although there is bilateral innervation of the upper one-third of the face, there is only one common path, in the lower motor neurone.

Upper motor neurone lesions

It is only on rare occasions that facial palsy is due to cortical lesion of the cerebral hemispheres, but can occur due to a focal lesion which may be moderately selective and cause a cerebral palsy. Most commonly facial palsy is seen as part of a hemiplegia due to haemorrhage or thrombosis in or around the internal capsule. Lesion of the ipsilateral temporal or frontal lobes can give rise to loss of emotional expression in the face. In contrast, this may be retained in patients with an upper motor neurone lesion which does not involve the frontal or temporal region. Understanding is far from complete regarding emotional expressions of the face. Subthalamic lesion involvement of the corpus striatum can give rise to poverty of facial expression, seen bilaterally in Parkinson's disease.

Lower motor neurone lesions

The lower motor neurone of the facial nerve starts with the facial nucleus in the pons, after fibres have crossed. In poliomyelitis the facial nucleus can rarely be involved as the sole feature of the disease. A correct diagnosis is usually only made during an epidemic and then there is a history of fever and malaise for some days before the palsy develops.

Before the facial nerve leaves the pons it may be involved in any pontine lesion. As there are a large number of tracts in close approximation in the pons the features may be diffuse with frequent bilateral or contralateral involvement. The sixth cranial nerve is often involved along with the seventh nerve and serves as a good localizing feature in facial palsy. Disseminated sclerosis may frequently involve the facial nerve, in which case the lesion is in the pons, subnuclear in position but not always involving the taste fibres. This type of facial palsy is usually transient and is associated with other neurological features which are in keeping with patchy demyelination. Pseudobulbar palsy can give facial weakness, sometimes of the upper motor neurone type with an increased jaw jerk.

The facial nerve as it leaves the pons in the cerebellopontine angle to enter the internal auditory canal can be compressed by an acoustic neuroma or even more rarely by a meningioma and basilar artery aneurysm. It is even possible on rare occasions for the facial nerve to be involved in this position in meningitis, usually of the chronic type or carcinomatosis, but even in these cases the facial nerve is not the only cranial nerve involved.

In the bony canal the facial nerve can be involved at various levels, due to tumours or infection. The level of involvement can be estimated as: below the geniculate ganglion where lacrimation will be spared, below the chorda tympani where taste from the anterior two-thirds of the tongue is spared or below the nerve to stapedius which, if involved, may give rise to hyperacusis due to fixation of the stapedius muscle.

The Ramsay-Hunt syndrome allegedly involves the facial nerve at the geniculate ganglion and Bell's palsy can involve the nerve anywhere in the bony canal, as can a fracture of the temporal bones of the skull. Haemorrhage may occur into the canal in hypertensive states and on rare occasions the nerve may be involved in various leukaemic and other malignant deposits. Lesions of the middle ear, like chronic otitis media and a cholesteatoma, can be rare causes of facial palsy, but the facial nerve is always in danger in ear surgery, especially in mastoidectomy.

After leaving the stylomastoid canal the nerve may be involved in parotid lesions. Benign tumours in the main displace the facial nerve, but malignant tumours involve the nerve and cause paralysis. Sarcoidosis of the parotid gland (as part of uveoparotitis) by its diffuse involvement of the gland can cause compression of the nerve with facial weakness. Traumatic use of forceps in delivery of an infant can cause facial paralysis which fortunately recovers in the majority of cases, but where it does not, the deformity can be very ugly with some lack of development of the facial muscles on the affected side. Stab wounds and facial lacerations, especially seen in patients involved in road traffic accicents while not wearing car safely belts, may also involve the facial nerve.

Any of the terminal branches may be involved in leprosy, but this is more common in the upper part of the face and can even be bilateral. It may be possible to palpate the nerve as a cord which c⁻n be rolled under the skin.

The facial nerve may be involved as part of an acute infective polyneuritis (Guillain–Barré syndrome). Like many of the conditions described where more diffuse neurological involvement occurs, the facial palsy becomes the last of the patient's problems in his fight for survival.

Myasthenia gravis, with its defective neuromuscular transmission, may first present as weakness of ocular movement or even facial movement that fatigues in speech.

Weakness of the facial muscles may be seen as part of any advanced case of any of the pure muscular dystrophies, but especially in the so-called facioscapular-humeral type; or similarly in any of the muscular dystrophies with myotonia, but again especially with dystrophia myotonica. The facioscapular-humeral muscular dystrophy is an autosomal dominant condition which is seen equally in the sexes and progresses very slowly. A dull-looking face which has no expression in conversation and can only just straighten the lips for a smile is characteristic, especially if seen with absence of blinking. As the name implies, the shoulders and upper part of the arms are also involved. Dystrophia myotonica is an autosomal dominant condition which is anticipated in each generation until it dies out. The first muscles involved are the sternomastoids and facial muscle, but the muscles of mastication may also be involved with progress to other muscle groups. Myotonic features are seen early in the disease before muscle wasting sets in. Other features of this condition are premature baldness, cataracts, testicular atrophy and cardiomyopathy developing in a high proportion of cases.

Incidence of facial palsy

It is hoped that the above account will dispel the idea that all cases of facial palsy are either Bell's palsy or part of a hemiplegia. Although these are by far the most common the rare condition will not be brought to light unless a full neurological examination, especially of the cranial nerves, is undertaken in all cases.

Cawthorne and Haynes (1956) reviewed the incidence of facial palsy, which was scored with a monthly index of 12 per 100 000 which makes it only slightly less frequent than thyrotoxicosis (14) and bronchiectasis (13). Of 557 cases of peripheral facial palsy reviewed, 347 were due to Bell's palsy, 84 due to injury, 39 to geniculate ganglion herpes, 27 infection, 22 neoplasm, 21 spasm, 11 nuclear and only 6 due to birth injury. In view of this more details will be given of Bell's palsy, geniculate herpes and facial muscular spasm, of which nothing has been said so far.

Bell's Palsy (Idiopathic Facial Palsy)

Named after Sir Charles Bell, the early nineteenth-century anatomist, this is the most common type of lower motor neurone facial palsy.

Aetiology

As the name implies, the aetiology of this condition is unknown. Although not proven it is often considered to be due to a virus infection.

With investigation of the Guillain–Barré syndrome, which is now thought to be due to allergic phenomena, interest has been shown in this mechanism as an aetiology for Bell's palsy but to date no antibodies have been detected. Ischaemia has also been postulated but not proven. Attempts have been made to localize the lesion; it would appear that 50 per cent are below the chorda tympani and the vast majority below the geniculate ganglion. There is no seasonal incidence nor are epidemics reported. Claims have been made for an abnormal appearance of the nerve as seen by bold surgeons.

Clinical features

Frequency is equal in the sexes and the condition can occur at almost any age on either side of the face, but not bilaterally. Recurrent attacks are recorded in about 10 per cent of cases. Bell's palsy develops quickly: often the patient awakens in the morning with a fully developed paralysis. There may be a preceding facial pain which is usually situated at the angle of the jaw. Very frequently the patient attributes his facial palsy to exposure to a cold wind.

In the majority of cases there is a palsy of the upper and lower parts of the face on the affected side. Some cases may have hyperacusis and in others there is loss of taste on the affected side while in rare cases there may be loss of lacrimation.

Taverner subdivided Bell's palsy into two groups according to electromyographical findings. An electrode was inserted at the angle of the jaw and the conduction time recorded between stimulation and twitching of the face.

1. *Conduction defect.* Here the conduction time never exceeds 4 msec. This is the milder of the two groups, with recovery starting in 2–21 days which is complete in 10–150 days with no sequels. This is seen in 60 per cent of cases of Bell's palsy.

2. *Denervation.* Here the conduction time is over 4 msec. Recovery does not start until about 7–150 days and may never be complete. This group accounts for 40 per cent of the cases of Bell's palsy with sequels occurring commonly, and 25 per cent of this group (10 per cent of the total) never recover.

Sequels of Bell's palsy

1. *Lacrimation:* This occurs in 15 per cent of cases where denervation is demonstrated. There is epiphora on the affected side either spontaneously or when the face is exposed to cold air.

2. *'Crocodile tears':* In 10 per cent of cases where there has been denervation this occurs, with tears streaming down the cheek as the patient eats. Amusing though this may sound, it is very distressing to the patient.

3. *Contracture of the muscles:* At first glance this may make the affected side appear normal but on close inspection it will be seen that this side does not move. This occurs frequently in cases with denervation and has been reported as almost 70 per cent in one series.

4. *Lack of recovery:* Usually even in the worst cases there is fortunately some recovery in the orbicularis oculi muscles. Although there may be many cases where recovery is incomplete when subjected to tests, only 10 per cent of all cases are finally dissatisfied with the result. This means that claims for successful treatment have to be evaluated very carefully and most have a success rate significantly higher than 90 per cent. The failure to realize this fact has led to many false claims for modes of treatment. It is in this condition perhaps more than any other that the value of well-controlled clinical trials are imperative.

Treatment

If the majority of cases are going to recover spontaneously, these patients are best treated conservatively with the main aim at protecting the eye until the muscle power starts to recover. Regular eye bathing is needed and some patients will need a temporary tarsorrhaphy. Patients are usually extremely distressed by the condition and want an active form of treatment. Many elaborate rituals have been devised, some involving elaborate apparatus and no doubt all able to claim a 90 per cent success rate. Simple massage of the face by the patient does no harm and may improve the patient's moral by making him think that he is achieving a useful cure. Logically, any treatment should be aimed at preventing sequelae and more specifically directed at the patients who do not spontaneously recover.

Cervical sympathetic block: Injection of the stellate ganglion with either alcohol or procaine has been advocated on the ground that the condition is due to ischaemia. There are no clinical trials which substantiate the effectiveness of this mode of treatment, and many authorities are doubtful of its use.

Surgical decompression of the facial nerve: A great wave of surgical bravado led to the drama of emergency decompression of the facial nerves, by removing the overlying bone. Allowing for surgical accidents, this is one of the few modes of treatment that does not have a 90 per cent success rate.

ACTH therapy: Taverner claimed that by giving ACTH early in the condition, cases which start as conduction blockade are not allowed to progress to denervation. The ACTH is given as follows:

Days 1–5	80 units
Day 6	60 units
Day 7	40 units
Day 8	20 units
Days 9 and 10	10 units

In a very convincing series Taverner showed that 76 out of 77 patients were completely cured. With these results it almost makes failure to treat early with ACTH negligence. Similar results may be achieved with prednisone which could be given orally, but understandably there is some hesitation to undertake a trial when such good results are already available. Since Taverner's original work, similar results have been achieved with a lower dose of ACTH starting at 40 or 60 units per day.

Dental treatment: Although hooks and slings have been found more nuisance than they have value, the dental surgeon still has his part to play. Patients may have difficulty with oral hygiene and in cases where there is some residual sagging of the face, a denture can be built out in the upper premolar and canine region to support the face.

Plastic surgery: Should be reserved for the cases where there is no recovery (this is considered later).

The Ramsay-Hunt Syndrome (Geniculate Herpes)

This is named after James Ramsay-Hunt, the neurologist from Boston, USA, who first described this condition in 1906. It is the only example of herpes apparently affecting a motor nerve, but it is as well to remember that the facial nerve is a mixed nerve.

Aetiology

There is no proof that the geniculate ganglion is involved, but serological tests have shown that *Herpes zoster* is responsible for the condition. The neurotropic properties of this virus are well known on sensory nerves.

Clinical features

For a few days before the herpetic eruption appears, there is a prodromal phase with fever, headache and malaise. There may even be preherpetic pain which can be localized to the ear or may radiate to the jaw and even down the neck. Occasionally, there is an area of hyperaesthesia.

Ramsay-Hunt classified the condition as follows:
  i. Herpetic oticus with no neurological signs.
  ii. As above with facial palsy.
  iii. As above with auditory signs.
  iv. As above with labyrinthine signs.

The zosteric eruption usually occurs a few days after the prodromal phase. There are small crops of vesicles which may appear on the tragus of the auricle or in the internal auditory meatus. Lesions occasionally occur on the tympanic membrane, which may perforate. The soft palate and the anterior two-thirds of the tongue may also be involved with facial eruptions occurring comparatively rarely. Associated with the eruption there may be pre- or post-auricular lymphadenopathy.

Facial palsy in the Ramsay-Hunt syndrome is unilateral of the lower motor neurone type which may appear at any time during the condition. In about 50 per cent of cases there is loss of taste on the affected side. There may be a unilateral perceptive deafness and possible labyrinthine features of tinnitus and vertigo. Post-herpetic pain is not a noted troublesome feature.

Course and prognosis

Complete recovery is usual but this may be delayed for up to two years, especially when the condition is seen in elderly patients.

Treatment

This is symptomatic as in Bell's palsy. The condition is too rare for good clinical trials using ACTH.

Clonic Facial Spasm

In this condition there are frequent involuntary contractions of facial muscles. As the condition is usually unilateral it is often called hemifacial spasm or, alternatively, facial myoclonia. The spasms are painless and the patient is unable to control their occurrence.

Aetiology

The aetiology is unknown but attempts have been made to divide the condition into:

1. *Symptomatic:* When the condition follows Bell's palsy or is associated with Ramsay-Hunt syndrome. Claims have been made for an associated between this condition and paroxysmal trigeminal neuralgia, but only in a few cases where the two have appeared at different times is the picture at all convincing.

2. *Cryptogenic:* Where no cause can be found, accounting for the majority of cases.

Clinical features

Clonic facial spasm is more common in females than it is in males and is rare in patients under the age of fifty years. It usually starts in the or-bicularis oculi muscles with twitching, and may spread to the lower part of the face. Only rarely is the condition seen bilaterally and then the spasm of the two sides are not synchronous. Gradually the condition mounts in its severity until the facial muscles are almost continuously in spasm. At this stage there is weakness of the facial musculature on the affected side and there may even be associated loss of taste.

The patient has no voluntary control of the spasms, which persist in sleep. Emotion and fatigue tend to make the condition worse.

It is rare for the condition to remit. Usually there is progression and the final ending is weakness and palsy. At no stage is the condition physically painful but there will be considerable psychological distress.

Differential diagnosis

Involuntary movements of the face are common but not all are clonic facial spasm. Twitching of the eyelids is a very common condition oc-curring in fatigued people of all ages. Habit spasms or tics are commonly seen in the face of children. It is possible for the child to control them for a time, but this is usually followed by a period of increased twitching. Often this type of condition is related to a personality disorder. Rather an unusual condition termed *maladie des tics*, Gilles de la Tourette's disease, facial tics and even almost continuous facial gestures are associated with involuntary expressions of foul language (echolalia). Eventually this condition progresses to schizophrenia.

Blepharospasm may be seen in patients with no apparent reason, but this is usually bilateral and is continuous spasm. Huntington's chorea can give facial spasm, but this, like athetosis, is associated with generalized muscular spasm.

Treatment

Surgical decompression of the nerve has not proved helpful but some cases have responded to mild trauma of the nerve as achieved by nipping it with forceps. Alcoholic injections into the nerve are a well tried remedy which can give relief for 6 months to 2 years, but this at the expense of a facial palsy. Faciohypoglossal anastomosis seems rather a radical procedure which could result in the loss of function of two cranial nerves, and is rightly falling from fashion. Claims have been made for carbamazepine (Tegretol), and this may well be worth a therapeutic trial before resorting to injection or surgical procedures.

Surgical Correction of Facial Palsy

A number of ingenious techniques have been undertaken by neuro- and plastic surgeons in an attempt to re-animate the lifeless face seen in facial palsy. It is only proposed to give the briefest summary.

Nerve grafts

Where the nerve has been sectioned, an attempt to join the two severed ends is the most logical approach. If a segment of nerve has been lost, nerve grafts have been undertaken using a variety of nerves which are relatively unimportant. Even the most enthusiastic authors describe only a 35 per cent improvement.

The anastomosis of intact nerves like the hypoglossal and accessory nerves to the distal portion of the facial nerve has been tried, but again the results are disappointing and there are further deformities from the donor site.

Fascial sling technique

Attempts have been made to support the facial muscles by wire slung from the zygoma, but this was abandoned in favour of strips of fascia lata. Two strips are often used, one joining the paralysed orbicularis oris muscles to those of the normal side and the second joining this strip of fascia to the zygoma or to the temporalis muscle. McLaughlin advocates drilling a hole in the coronoid process of the mandible fixing the fascia to the bone and then to cut the coronoid process off, so that the fascia is effectively joined to the temporalis muscle. In the right hands this type of operation enjoys reasonable success.

Face lift

Other surgeons have tried to correct the facial sagging by cosmetic plastic surgery.

Muscle transplants

Ambitious attempts have been made to use the anterior part of the masseter muscle by inserting it into the angle of the mouth, or even the sternocleidomastoid muscle. Both these muscle techniques are rather clumsy and give results inferior to the fascial sling techniques.

Bibliography

Brain W. R. (1962) *Diseases of the Nervous System.* 6th ed. London, Oxford University Press.

Cawthorne T. and Haynes D. R. (1956) Facial palsy. *Br. Med. J.* 2, 1197.

Cohen L. (1967) Hemifacial spasm. *Oral Surg.* 23, 592.

Conway H. (1958) Muscle plastic operations for facial paralysis. *Ann. Surg.* 147, 541.

McLaughlin C. R. (1952) Permanent facial paralysis, the role of surgical support. *Lancet* 2, 647.

Miller H. (1967) Facial paralysis. *Br. Med. J.* 3, 815.

Nally F. F. (1970) Melkersson-Rosanthal syndrome. *Oral Surg.* 29, 694.

Patey D. H. (1963) Risk of facial paralysis after parotidectomy. *Br. Med. J.* 2, 1100.

Taverner D. (1959) The prognosis and treatment of spontaneous facial palsy. *Proc. R. Soc. Med.* 52, 1077.

Taverner D. (1964) The treatment of facial palsy. *Practitioner* 192, 78.

Taverner D. *et al.* (1966) Prevention of denervation in Bell's palsy. *Br. Med. J.* 1, 391.

Chapter 20

Cervicofacial Lymphadenopathy

Over a quarter of the lymph nodes in the body are situated in the head and the neck. It is not surprising then, that many diseases of the lymphoid tissue present primarily in this region.

Anatomy (Fig. 7)

Lymph drainage from the superficial tissue of the head and neck generally goes in the first instance to groups of superficially placed lymph nodes, before passing to the deep cervical lymph nodes. In the occipital region there are a few lymph nodes which drain the posterior part of the scalp. The parietal region of the scalp drains to the mastoid lymph nodes, while the external ear and the region of the angle of the jaw drain to the superficial cervical lymph nodes which are found superficial to the upper part of the sternomastoid muscle. Lymph from the temporal region of the scalp drains into the superficial parotid lymph nodes. The lateral part of the frontal region, the middle ear and the lateral part of the eye lids also drain into the parotid lymph nodes. From the medial part of the frontal region, the medial part of the eye lid and the skin of the nose, cheek and upper lip, lymphatics follow the anterior facial vein to end in the submandibular lymph nodes. The lower lip drains into the submental lymph nodes, but often the lateral part drains to the submandibular lymph nodes.

All the groups of the lymph nodes so far mentioned drain into the deeper cervical lymph nodes. Most of the deeper structures drain straight into this same lymph chain. There are other groups of lymph nodes in the neck, which surround the larynx, pharynx and trachea. Only those lymph nodes draining the mouth and associated structures will be considered.

The gums and teeth of the lower jaw together with the floor of the mouth drain to the submandibular lymph nodes. Maxillary teeth, gums and hard palate drain straight to the deep cervical lymph nodes, while the soft palate drains to the retropharyngeal and deep cervical lymph nodes.

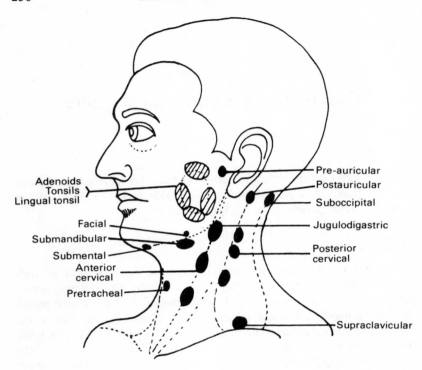

Adenoids
Tonsils
Lingual tonsil

Facial
Submandibular
Submental
Anterior
cervical
Pretracheal

Pre-auricular
Postauricular
Suboccipital
Jugulodigastric
Posterior
cervical
Supraclavicular

Fig. 7. Position of lymph nodes of the head and neck

There is a lymphatic plexus within the tongue with the tip of the tongue draining to the submental lymph nodes, the rest of the anterior two thirds to the submandibular nodes and the posterior third direct to the upper part of the deep cervical chain. In the midline there is some cross-over of lymphatic drainage from one side to the other.

Tonsillar lymph drains into the jugulodigastric lymph node and upper part of the deep cervical chain. It must be remembered that the tonsil is lymphoid tissue itself and may be involved in lymphadenopathy, as for example lymphosarcoma. In addition to the tonsil there is tonsillar material in the posterior aspect of the tongue and the posterior wall of the pharynx. These three form a ring of lymphoid tissue round the oropharynx. If all are involved dysphagia is experienced.

Examination

Quite often the patient is aware that he has a lymphadenopathy, usually covered by the lay term 'glands in the neck'. Tenderness may have drawn the patient's attention to their presence, but there are some who seem to have an obsession for examining themselves, and will find the most minute of lumps which even the skilled clinician has difficulty in discovering.

Most of the examination, after a quick front and side facial inspection for obvious deformity, is undertaken from behind the seated patient. This should be the rule regardless of the patient being in bed or ambulant. Systematically, each region needs to be examined lightly with the pulps of the fingers, trying to roll the lymph nodes against harder underlying structures. Parotid, mastoid and occipital lymph nodes can be palpated simultaneously using both hands. To examine submental lymph nodes the patient's head is best tipped forward and the lymph nodes rolled against the inner aspect of the mandible. Submandibular lymph nodes are examined in the same way with the patient's head tipped to the side which is being examined. Differentiation needs to be made between the submandibular salivary gland and submandibular lymph glands. This can be very difficult as lymph nodes may be buried in the substance of the salivary gland. Bimanual examination with one finger in the floor of the mouth may help. Examination of the deep cervical lymph chain is always incomplete as only the lymph nodes which project anterior or posterior to the sternomastoid muscle can be palpated. For the few glands that can be palpated in this region, there must be many more under the muscle. It is not often that the thyroid gland causes confusion, but nodules in the thyroid gland may be temporarily misleading, until the patient is asked to swallow, and the lump moves with the thryoid gland. A search for the jugulodigastric lymph node should be specifically undertaken, as this is the most common lymph node involved in tonsillar infections.

Superficial cervical lymph nodes need to be examined with lighter fingers as they can only be compressed against the softer sternomastoid muscle. Paralaryngeal and tracheal lymph nodes can be compressed lightly against the trachea. The supraclavicular region should be examined at the same time as the rest of the neck, lymph nodes here may extend up into the posterior triangle of the neck on the scalene muscles, behind the sternomastoid.

No examination of the lymphatics of the head and neck is complete without inspection of the tonsils. Strictly speaking, all the tonsillar ring should be examined, the oropharyngeal, nasopharyngeal and lingual tonsil, but for most examinations inspection of the oropharyngeal tonsil will suffice.

Some information can be gained by the texture and nature of the lymphadenopathy. Note should be made of single or multiple lymph nodes, and if the occurrence is unilateral or bilateral. The consistency is also important, and is best described under three headings: soft, firm and hard. Attention should also be paid to whether the nodes are fixed to each other, often called 'matted', fixed to skin and deeper structures, or free and mobile. Tenderness and swelling should also be documented.

Lymph nodes from acute infections are usually tender, soft and discrete, while chronic infections give firm lymph nodes. Secondary malignancy gives hard fixed glands and malignant lymphomas give firm matted lymph nodes, in multiple sites. The tip of the cricoid cartilage may be mistaken for a hard gland, while the carotid sinus or even a sebaceous cyst may mimic soft lymph nodes.

It goes without saying that where there are a number of lymph nodes palpated in the head and neck, other sites must be inspected for lymphadenopathy, hepatomegaly, and splenomegaly. A chest X-ray will show hilar lymphadenopathy, which can be a distressing cause of dyspnoea.

Causes of Lymphadenopathy

Local infections

This is one of the commonest causes of lymphadenopathy. Any infection will cause some congestion of the local lymphatics, not always to the degree of giving discrete lymphadenopathy. In acute infections there may just be tenderness in the area of the regional lymph nodes, rather than definite palpable lymph nodes. A more chronic infection gives discernible lymph node enlargement.

Most chronic lesions of the mouth give a lymphadenopathy in the submandibular region. Even conditions like aphthous ulcers and pericoronitis may produce lymphatic involvement. The fact that the primary lesion was not infective in origin makes little difference, as secondary infection in the mouth is almost invariable.

Superficial infections of the scalp can cause enlarged lymph nodes in the occipital, mastoid or parotid region. Infection of the middle ear can be the origin of deep cervical lymphadenopathy, and tonsillitis the source of enlarged jugulodigastric lymph nodes. Diphtheria is noted for its 'bull neck' appearance, which is due to a lymphadenopathy.

Tuberculous lymphadenitis

This was a once common condition, as evidenced by the number of scars seen on the necks of middle-aged people. With the advent of compulsory tuberculosis testing of cattle in the United Kingdom, the condition has become almost extinct. Cervical lymphadenopathy was one of the most common sites of tuberculous lymphadenopathy, with 70 per cent occurring in the upper deep cervical glands anterior to the sternomastoid, but they could occur in the posterior triangle of the neck and even low in the anterior part. The involved node could caseate and break down to form the so-called 'collar stud abscess', which discharged from a sinus in the neck.

Usually the infection was from the bovine type of tubercule, which gained access through the tonsil or pharynx. Generally the infection occurred in infancy, but adults were sometimes affected. The condition is wont to follow a subacute form with some pain and swelling in the neck. On other occasions tuberculosis is chronic, with the formation of the so-called 'abscess'. In all cases the Mantoux test is strongly positive at a dilution of 1:10 000. Treatment consists of a combined chemotherapeutic and surgical approach.

Syphilitic lymphadenopathy

Cervical lymphadenopathy can occur for various reasons in syphilis. In the rare event of the primary chancre being oral there will be a rubbery lymphadenopathy in the submandibular and even cervical regions. In secondary syphilis there may be a generalized lymphadenopathy, and this will nearly always involve the cervical region. Mucosal ulcers ('snail track patches') of the mouth can give rise to a submandibular lymphadenopathy and there will generally be a lymphadenopathy when a gumma is found in the mouth. Diagnosis of syphilis is made by confirmatory serological tests, but not all lymphadenopathies with positive syphilitic serology are due to syphilis.

Infectious mononucleosis (glandular fever)

This is a common benign disease which is now recognized to have many forms, but often takes the form of a febrile lymphadenopathy, as its name implies. It is more fully considered in Chapter 3.

Acquired toxoplasmosis

This is a protozoal infection, more fully considered in Chapter 4 in which cervical lymphadenopathy is a common presentation.

Cat-scratch fever

Rare though this condition is, scratches on the head and neck are common enough from fondling a cat. The type of lymphadenopathy is fairly non-specific, but might break down with abscess formation. Even in the absence of suppuration the condition may take several months to subside. Any treatment is non-specific as the infecting agent has not been identified.

The histiocytoses

This represents a rare group of conditions which, although not necessarily related, are best mentioned together. Eosinophilic granuloma, Schüller–Christian disease, Letterer–Siwe disease, Gaucher's disease and Niemann–Pick disease can all cause lymphadenopathy. Often the diagnosis can only be made by histology of a biopsied lymph node.

Sarcoidosis

This may present as a benign lymphogranulomatosis, but may also involve almost any organ of the body.

Lymphadenopathy, especially in the cervical region, together with arthritis and erythema nodosa are common primary manifestations.

Sarcoid has a world wide distribution but occurs slightly more frequently in Sweden than other countries. In the United Kingdom the incidence is 20 per 100 000. The condition is most commonly seen in women of child-bearing age. Irish and West Indians, for some unknown reason, have a higher incidence when living in England or the United States of America.

Aetiology: No cause has been found for sarcoid, although many interesting theories have been put forward. These range from infection to auto-immunity, and include chemical hypersensitivity and reticuloendothelial overactivity.

Clinical features: There are two forms of this disease which overlap. An acute type, which may remit completely or pass on to the second type of the disease, which is more chronic and permanent in character. Cervical lymphadenopathy may occur in both, but is more discrete in the first and forms with diffuse fibrosis in the second. Hilar lymphadenopathy is most commonly seen, and may be spotted on routine chest X-ray.

The patient usually has a mild fever and feels generally unwell with gradual loss of weight. The lungs are diseased most commonly of many possible sites involved, with lymph nodes next in frequency. It is not proposed here to discuss the complications of involvement of other organs of the body and their clinical manifestations. The clinical features of involvement of the mucosa of the oral cavity and of salivary glands are covered in Chapters 10 and 12.

In brief, the acute form carries a good prognosis while the chronic form, although more insidious, has a higher morbidity and mortality rate.

Diagnosis: In the initial phase the ESR will be raised, often associated with increased alpha and gammaglobulin. The white cell count is usually slightly raised, possibly with some degree of eosinophilia and monocytosis. Alternatively, there may be leucopenia, anaemia and thrombocytopenia. Elevation of the serum calcium is always significant and will fall rapidly after the administration of steroids. Biopsy may also be helpful. Two-thirds of patients with sarcoid have a negative Mantoux test. The specific test for sarcoid is the Kveim test, in which a saline suspension of an extract of a lymph node of a patient with active sarcoid is injected subcutaneously. A cutaneous red nodule develops, which is biopsied after six weeks and shows the appearance of a sarcoid granuloma.

Treatment: Often the best treatment is bed rest and observation. There are set criteria for the administration of steroids: these include eye involvement, persistent chest features with breathlessness, neurological features, involvement of salivary or lacrimal glands, hypercalcaemia, severe skin or mucosal lesions and the rare involvement of the heart. Salicylates, phenylbutazone and even chloroquinine derivatives have a place in selected cases.

Lymphoreticular Neoplasms

Hodgkin's Disease (Lymphadenoma): This is yet another lymphatic disease of unknown origin. Diagnosis is dependent on finding the Reed–Sternberg multinucleated giant cells on histology of the lymph nodes. Hodgkin's disease is usually accepted as being neoplastic, but a viral cause cannot be ruled out.

Clinical features

Men are twice as commonly affected as women, and most cases occur in the 20–40 age group. Cervical lymphadenopathy is often the first sign, but Hodgkin's disease has an 'iceberg' feature: the lymph nodes that can be palpated represent only a small proportion of the total lymph nodes involved. Thus, often the clinical finding of cervical lymphadenopathy is followed by a chest X-ray which shows invasion of mediastinal lymph nodes. Any group of lymph nodes may be affected and the spleen enlarged. Other organs outside the reticuloendothelial system can also be involved, but often the symptoms are produced by presence of lymph node enlargement.

The patient generally feels unwell, with anorexia and loss of weight. Lymphadenopathy appears quickly, the lymph nodes being discrete, rubbery in consistency and painless. As the patient often complains of a sore throat the lymphadenopathy is often excused on local grounds in the first instance. Pruritus is a noticeable troublesome feature in about a quarter of patients. There may be nodular skin lesions common on the face or scalp. Ulcers of a non-specific type often occur in the mouth. Often there is a fever, even with night sweats. The fever may remit for short periods to return again at rising levels over several days and then fall again; this is known as the Pel–Ebstein fever, with a compatible tachycardia.

There is a strange feature in Hodgkin's disease which is only rarely seen in other malignant disease; that is of pain in the areas involved by Hodgkin's disease after the ingestion of even small quantities of alcohol. This feature remits with effective treatment.

Patients are often anaemic, which may be haemolytic in type. This is not usually enough to make the patient jaundiced, but with liver involvement jaundice may occur.

Haematological findings

In no way diagnositic, but the anaemia may be Coomb's positive and there may be a leucocytosis or even a leucopenia. In 12 per cent of cases there will be an eosinophilia.

Course and prognosis

This is very variable and depends on the rapidity of the condition. Some patients live for more than 20 years, while others are dead within 6 months. The rapidly fatal type is often called Hodgkin's sarcoma and the very slow type Hodgkin's paragranuloma. Perhaps more satisfactory is the system of typing according to the degree of spread. Cases with only lymph nodes in one region have the best prognosis, while patients with widespread dissemination and systemic features have a poor prognosis.

Complications

Of the many complications to this disease, the most important from the oral point of view is the patient's susceptibility to infection, especially viral and gungal. Oral candidosis is common and so is *herpes zoster.*

Diagnosis

This is a differential from any other lymphadenopathy and the only way to make a sure diagnosis is by biopsy. Early involvement of lymph nodes may not give a characteristic appearance, and so the largest available lymph node gives the best result; even then it may be necessary to repeat the biopsy on more than one occasion.

Treatment

Opinions differ on the best way to treat Hodgkin's disease. If the glands are purely localized, the patients respond well to deep X-ray therapy. The problem is to know if glands are involved in other parts of the body. Most clinicians would prefer to give some form of chemotherapy as well. Nitrogen mustard is initially very effective given intravenously. If this fails cyclophosphamide, chlorambucil or ibenzmethazine should be tried.

Supportive treatment may be needed, such as blood transfusions for the anaemia. Steroids may help to prevent haemolytic anaemia.

Lymphosarcoma and Reticulosarcoma: These are two neoplastic conditions of lymph nodes that are best considered together as differentiation is purely academic, since the two conditions have a similar course. Nothing is known of the aetiology. Both occur in a wide age group, but become more frequent in older patients.

Clinical features

Once again cervical lymphadenopathy may be the first manifestation. Not infrequently the tonsils are involved early in the disease, being grossly augmented and often meeting in the midline. Other lymph nodes are rapidly affected and spreading occurs to other organs more quickly than with Hodgkin's disease. Cutaneous manifestations are not so often seen, but *herpes zoster* and oral candidosis are common. Involvement of the central nervous system may give rise to cranial nerve palsy. A Horner's syndrome may be caused by compression of the cervical sympathetic chain.

Diagnosis

This is always by lymph node biopsy. Late in the disease there may be spill-over of cells into the blood stream, which gives a clinical picture of lymphatic leukaemia, even the bone marrow may be involved in the same way.

Treatment and prognosis

Radiotherapy to local lesions cause an initial good response but this is short lived. Cytotoxic drugs, especially cyclophosphamide, can give some clinical improvement, but the prognosis is extremely poor with few patients living for more than two years.

Brill–Symmer's Disease (Giant Follicular Lymphoma): This is only mentioned for the sake of completeness. There is serious question if this disease has a right to be classed as a disease. It has many features in common with the lymphasarcoma, and others in common with Hodgkin's disease. Often the condition settles to follow the course of either Hodgkin's disease or lymphosarcoma. Diagnosis is only made on biopsy and treatment is by radiotherapy and chemotherapy.

Lymphadenopathy in Leukaemias: About a third of acute leukaemias present as a lymphadenopathy. Chronic lymphatic leukaemia most commonly presents with lymph node enlargement.

Acute leukaemias

Characteristically seen in children who may appear pale, tired and listless. As pyrexia is frequent, it is easy to assume that the child has an infectious disease, especially as there is often an upper respiratory infection. The infective element in itself leads to a lymphadenopathy, with lymph nodes which may be tender and inflamed. Cervical lymphadenopathy is not the solitary reticular involvement, other lymph nodes and even the liver and spleen may be enlarged.

Bleeding tendencies are very common, they may take the form of ecchymoses or petechial haemorrhages. There may be frank bleeding from the gums or the nose. Often the gums are swollen and inflamed even to the point of teeth disappearing beneath a mass of hyperplastic spongy gingival tissue. Oral features are notorious in monocytic leukaemia where the gums may be stuffed with leukaemia cells. Large, painful, infected and non-specific ulcers complete the misery of acute monocytic leukaemia.

Secondary involvement of bones and joints and even of the nervous system are common. Almost any organ can be involved which may be damaged by the leukaemic deposits or there may be haemorrhage or sepsis.

Diagnosis

This is by haematological investigation, where the abnormal cells can be seen. Rarely will marrow puncture be necessary, lymph node biopsy not being the usual way of making the diagnosis. Thus in all cases of lymphadenopathy it is as well to await the result of haematology before proceeding to biopsy.

Bleeding is due to the thrombocytopenia which occurs. Anaemia may be marked and is not helped by haemorrhage.

Treatment

After transfusion, the current line of treatment in children is steroids and rotational cytotoxic drugs.

Chronic Leukaemia: Lymphadenopathy is most frequently seen in chronic lymphatic leukaemia but is by no means rare in chronic myloid leukaemia. Chronic lymphatic leukaemia is a disease repeatedly seen in old men, chronic myeloid leukaemia covers a wide age span. As the disease develops insidiously the patient may notice a group of lymph nodes or may feel generally unwell. Routine investigation of some other disease may bring to light a chronic leukaemia. Other lymphoid tissue is commonly involved and enlarged tonsils might be seen in chronic lymphatic leukaemia; hepatosplenomegaly is common to both diseases. Chronic myeloid leukaemia is one of the few causes of gross splenomegaly.

Again almost any organ can be involved with leukaemic deposits but this is not so familiar as in the acute leukaemias. Skin lesions are quite common and may take the form of nodular deposits or the rare but well known, generalized reddening of the skin known as 'l'homme rouge'.

Terminally both leukaemias can take an acute form with haemorrhage and anaemia being prominent.

Complications

Vaccination for smallpox is contraindicated as there is a definite danger of vaccinia gangrenosa. Herpes zoster and oral candidosis are besetting complications.

Diagnosis

Usually possible from a blood film, but a marrow puncture is an established court of appeal. Anaemia may not be a prominent feature of early chronic leukaemia. There may be a positive Coomb's test with a possible haemolytic anaemia especially in lymphatic leukaemia. In myloid leukaemia the red cells do not stain well for alkaline phosphatase and the serum vitamin B_{12} level may be over 1000 micrograms per millilitre. The serum uric acid may be raised, but not so regularly as in acute leukaemias.

Treatment

Busulphan is the drug of choice for chronic myeloid leukaemia and Chlorambucil for chronic lymphatic leukaemia. Often old patients with mild chronic lymphatic leukaemia are best left untreated as the disease may remain static or be very slow in progress with the patients living many years before they die of some totally unrelated disease. Anaemia will need treatment with blood transfusions, but if there is a haemolytic element to the case steroids will increase the length of time between transfusions.

Secondary Malignancies: Carcinoma metastasizes via the lymphatics, so one of the first signs that a carcinoma is spreading is for the regional lymph nodes to be involved. The group of lymph nodes involved depends on the site of the primary tumour. Tumours of the mouth and tongue metastasize to the submandibular, sublingual and cervical lymph nodes.

On palpation the lymph nodes are hard and generally fixed to the surrounding tissues. Usually it is possible to find the primary site, but occasionally cervicofacial lymphadenopathy is the first manifestation of the malignancy. On these occasions a biopsy of the lymph node may help to determine the primary site.

In the case of malignant ulcers of the mouth, the presence of lymphadenopathy is not always significant of spread. It is common for the primary ulcer to become infected and this will give rise to a lymphadenopathy. If this is the case the lymph nodes will be soft, discrete and tender. Unfortunately, both processes may go on together so this sign cannot be relied on.

As a general rule metastases in the anterior triangle of the neck are from tongue, mouth, pharynx, larynx, oesophagus or thyroid. Posterior triangle metastases are usually from stomach, pancreas, bronchus, breast or oesophagus.

Other Cases of Lymphadenopathy: In a number of diseases a lymphadenopathy is part of the disorder. To make mention of all the diseases which have associated lymphadenopathy would prolong this section beyond reason. Thus it will have to suffice to mention a few diseases where lymphadenopathy is a prominent feature. In rubella it is commonplace to find an occipital lymphadenopathy. Other acute fevers may be associated with lymphadenopathy. Patients with rheumatoid or systemic lupus erythematosus will frequently have palpable lymph glands. Thyrotoxicosis and even diabetes may be associated with lymph node enlargement. Epileptics treated with sodium phenytoin sporadically have lymphadenopathy.

There are some patients who are completely well in every aspect, but have persistent lymphadenopathy. It is debatable if there is any value in subjecting them to lymph node biopsy provided they have a normal blood picture and no elevation of the ESR.

References

Beverley J. K. A. and Beattie C. P. (1958) Glandular toxoplasmosis. *Lancet* 2, 379.
British Medical Journal (1969) 3, 190. Leading Article, 'More about glandular fever.'
Edmond R. T. D. (1968) Infectious mononucleosis. *Hosp. Med.* 2, 1084.
James D. G. (1967) Clinical aspects of sarcoid. *Hosp. Med.* 2, 8.
Ramsay A. M. and Edmond R. T. D. (1967) *Infectious Diseases*. London, Heinemann.
Thompson R. B. (1965) *Short Textbook of Haematology*, 2nd ed. London, Pitman.
Tidy, Sir Henry (1952) Glandular fever. *Br. Med. J.* 2, 436.
Walls E. W. (1964) in Cunningham's *Textbook of Anatomy*, 10th ed. London, Oxford University Press.

Chapter 21

Metabolic Bone Disease

Introduction

Calcium, phosphate and bone are inextricably linked and metabolic bone disease is taken to include disturbances in calcium and phosphate metabolism which have an effect upon bones. These disturbances result from aberrations in absorption or excretion of calcium and phosphate due to diseases of the gut or kidney (or dietary deficiency of the ions), or of the mechanisms controlling intermediary metabolism.

It is customary to include some disorders of unknown aetiology but here only Paget's disease will be noted from that group. It is obvious that many inherited diseases involving the skeleton are due to metabolic aberrations involving bone but they will not be considered here.

There are only two basic skeletal expressions of metabolic bone disease—they are osteoporosis and osteomalacia. In osteoporosis the total volume of bone tissue in the body is reduced but whatever bone remains is normally calcified (brittle bones). In osteomalacia the total volume of bone tissue is normal (or increased) but much of that tissue is poorly calcified (soft bones). (*Fig.* 8.)

Osteitis fibrosa, as seen in hyperparathyroidism, consists of osteoporosis with the lost bone replaced by fibrous tissue. The bone shows active resorption with osteoclasts.

Physiology

In the normal adult 99 per cent of body calcium and phosphate are crystallized in bone tissue upon which they confer rigidity. The 1 per cent of each ion outside bone have very important properties. Intracellular calcium is involved in mediating intracellular events following surface activation in nerves, muscles and other cells. The effects of calcium are profoundly influenced by the extracellular concentration of the ion and so there are extremely effective mechanisms for keeping that concentration

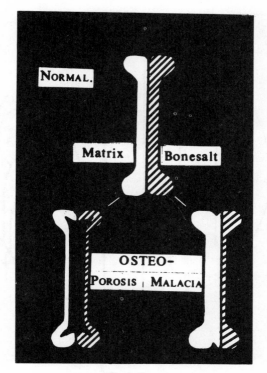

NORMAL.

Matrix Bonesalt

OSTEO-
POROSIS | MALACIA

Fig. 8. *See* text.

within very strict limits.

The normal serum calcium is 10 mg (9–11)/100 ml; (2·1–2·6 mmol/l). It exists in three forms:

—ionized (50 per cent) 5 mg/100 ml.

—protein bound (40 per cent) 4 mg/100 ml.

—complexed (10 per cent) 1 mg/100 ml.

The proportion bound to protein varies directly with the serum albumin while the ionized portion varies inversely with serum pH.

The serum phosphate is 2–4 mg/100 ml (0·6–1·40 mmol/l).

The serum calcium and phosphate tend to vary inversely but their product is very constant and in normality always exceeds 40 mg/100 ml.

In the normal adult in calcium balance about 1000 mg are taken by mouth per day, and 1000 mg are lost in faeces and urine; 100 mg net are absorbed from the gut into the extracellular pool, which is in equilibrium with bone, and from that pool 100 mg are lost in the urine (*Fig.* 9).

This external balance disguises large fluxes between the extracellular pool

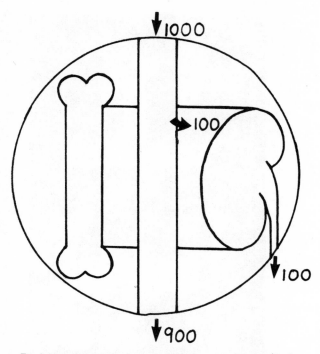

Fig. 9. External calcium balance in the normal adult (mg/day).

and the bone calcium which represents 99 per cent of ion in the body (*Fig.* 10).

Bone matrix may be regarded as having a high affinity for calcium so that when there is net production of matrix, for instance in growth, the serum calcium tends to be 'lowered' by deposition into bone and mechanisms come into play involving vitamin D and its renal metabolites, and parathormone (*vide infra*), to enhance absorption from the gut.

Bone salt when first deposited has a Ca:P ratio of 8:6, i.e. $Ca_8H_2(PO_4)_6$ octacalcium hexaphosphate.

Mature bone salt however is hydroxyapatite with a Ca:P ratio of 10:6, i.e. $Ca_{10}(OH)_2(PO_4)_6$.

Calcium and phosphate are supersaturated in serum so that bone powder placed in serum absorbs calcium and phosphate from the serum during equilibration. However, spontaneous crystallization of octacalcium hexaphosphate will only take place at much higher product concentrations of the ions than that found in normal plasma.

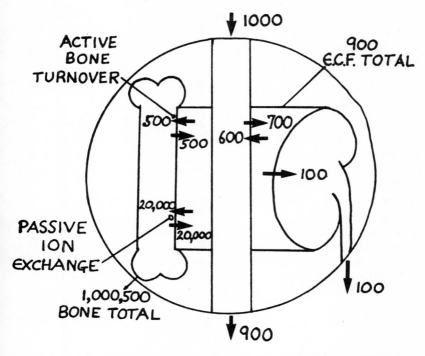

Fig. 10. Calcium fluxes between the bone, extracellular fluid, gut and kidney in the normal adult (mg/day).

The role of bone matrix and cellular activity must, therefore, be crucial in ossification but the detailed biochemical events are unknown.

Vitamin D and parathormone are known to promote resorption of bone (*vide infra*). How this is achieved is unknown but is mediated through osteoclasts. It is known that some prostaglandins can promote bone resorption and they may be significant at the edges of soft-tissue lesions in bones, such as cysts and tumours. Whether the prostaglandins stimulate osteoclasts or whether they are part of the normal mechanism operated by osteoclasts is not known.

Calcium absorption from the gut is diminished by reduced need and excess phosphate and phytate in the diet.

Parathormone: This is a protein, with 84 amino acids, of which secretion is stimulated by low serum calcium. The 'normal' serum concentration is less than 1 ng/1. The hormone has four actions, three of which directly cause a rise in the serum calcium (*Fig.* 11):

a. It diminishes phosphate resorption by renal tubules, with resulting phosphaturia.

b. It enhances calcium resorption by the renal tubules, retaining calcium.

c. It promotes solution of bone by enhancing osteoclastic activity, causing hypercalcaemia; the released phosphate is lost by action (*a*).

d. It stimulates renal 1α-hydroxylase which causes production of 1, 25-$(OH)_2$ cholecalciferol, the most active renal metabolite (hormone) of vitamin D. This in turn promotes absorption of calcium from the gut and has identical actions (*b*), (*c*), as parathormone.

Parathormone is metabolized by the kidney.

Vitamin D: The diet provides a fat-soluble cholecalciferol, which may also be produced in the skin by the action of sunlight on endogenous dehydrocholesterol. Cholecalciferol (Vitamin D_3), is oxidized in the liver to 25-hydroxycholecalciferol $(25,OH,D_3)$ which is a 'prohormone', further metabolized in the kidney. In the presence of a normal serum

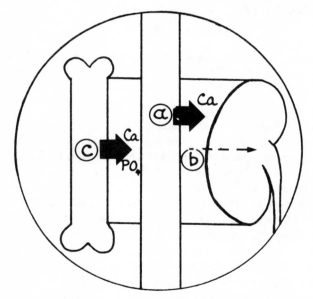

Fig. 11. The actions of parathormone: (*a*) Enhanced phosphate excretion. (*b*) Diminished calcium excretion. (*c*) Bone solution. (*d*) Promotion of 1α-hydroxylase.

calcium and phosphate (low or absent circulating parathormone) the kidney converts the prohormone into 24,25-dihydroxycholecalciferol $(24,25(OH)_2D_3)$ and 1,24,25-trihydroxycholecalciferol $(1,24,25(OH)_3D_3)$ which are weakly active. When the serum calcium is low and parathormone secretion is high renal 1α-hydroxylase activity is enhanced and the prohormone is converted to 1,25-dihydroxycholecalciferol $(1,25(OH)_2D_3)$ which is the most active form. Production of this hormone may also be enhanced by low serum phosphate.

The renal hormones derived from vitamin D_3 have, in varying degrees, the following actions (*Fig.* 12):

a. Promote calcium absorption from the gut.

b. Enhance calcium resorption by the renal tubules, diminishing calcium excretion.

c. Stimulate solution of calcium and phosphate from bone.

(*b*) and (*c*) are identical to two actions of parathormone.

All the actions of vitamin D tend to cause hypercalcaemia.

Although vitamin D causes solution of bone its principal action is to promote absorption of calcium from the gut and so make it available for calcification. The lytic action is more than balanced by the absorption of calcium from the gut and renal retention (*Fig.* 12).

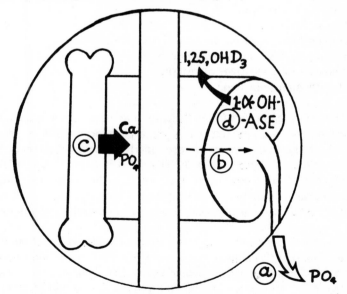

Fig. 12. The actions of vitamin D: (*a*) Promotes adsorption of calcium from gut. (*b*) Reduces calcium excretion. (*c*) Promotes solution of bone salt.

Vitamin D is metabolized in the liver.

Calcitonin: This is a 32 amino acid peptide produced by the parafollicular (c) cells of the thyroid. It is probably secreted regularly since its life is short. It inhibits resorption of bone and enhances bone deposition by osteoblasts. Thus it tends to lower serum calcium.

The diseases associated with disturbed calcium metabolism may be classified as follows:

1. DISTURBANCES OF CALCIUM HOMOEOSTASIS WITH RESULTANT EFFECT UPON BONE MINERALIZATION

    a. Dietary deficit—calcium.
    b. Vitamin D deficiency.
    c. Vitamin D excess.
    d. Abnormal vitamin D metabolism; liver and renal tubular disease.
    e. Hyperparathyroidism.
    f. Hypoparathyroidism.
    g. Uraemia.

2. OSTEOPOROSIS

    a. Steroid hormones.
    b. Pituitary hormones.
    c. Thyroid hormones.
    d. Senile osteoporosis.

3. DISEASES CAUSING BONE DESTRUCTION

    a. Carcinomatosis and myelomatosis.

4. DISORDERS OF UNKNOWN AETIOLOGY

    a. Paget's disease of bone.

1(*a*). *Dietary calcium deficiency.* Calcium may be deficient in the diet or may be combined with phytate which prevents absorption, but in practice these are unimportant, except in the elderly. Osteomalacia may be a significant factor in bone loss in the elderly; it is found in up to 30 per cent of patients with femoral neck fracture. In malabsorption syndromes calcium malabsorption may lead to deficiency but it is more likely to be secondary to the associated steatorrhoea with loss of dietary vitamin D.

1(*b*). *Vitamin D deficiency* may result from an inadequate diet but in advanced countries usually results from reduced absorption due to steatorrhoea. In unpigmented people in good sunlight this can be compensated for by production of vitamin D_3 in the skin so that resulting disease in sunless England is commoner in immigrants.

As a result of diminished body vitamin D, from whatever cause, there is a reduction in gut calcium absorption and a tendency to lowered serum calcium. This in turn results in parathormone secretion and diversion of vitamin D metabolism to production of the most active hormone, $1,25(OH)_2D_3$.

The parathormone secretion causes phosphaturia with hypophosphataemia but a relatively normal serum calcium. New bone matrix is poorly calcified with overall net loss of bone tissue. Clinically rickets results in children and osteomalacia in adults.

In rickets and osteomalacia there is invariably a low plasma Ca x P product. In most cases this is due to a marked fall in phosphate and a low or low-normal calcium. The Ca x P in normals is 40 and in rickets 30 (values between 30 and 40 are equivocal). The alkaline phosphatase is raised. Urinary calcium is low while urinary phosphate may be normal due to low plasma phosphate due to hyperparathyroidism.

Pathology: The whole skeleton is diminished in bulk. The major effect is upon ossification in cartilage with enlargement of the epiphysial plate with disorderly vascularization, defective calcification of cartilage and excess of osteoid.

After epiphyseal closure, in adults, osteomalacia results in the formation of excess (uncalcified) osteoid. Osteoid borders are thickened but more significantly extend over a greater surface of bone trabeculae than normal (upper limit of normal 26 per cent).

In addition there may be histological evidence of hyperparathyroidism (osteitis fibrosa and excess osteoclasts).

Vitamin deficiency may be corrected by giving 1000 i.u. daily by mouth. If due to malabsorption, intramuscular injection if necessary.

1(c). *Vitamin D,* given in excess, leads to enhanced calcium absorption and hypercalcaemia. There tends to be extraosseous (metastatic) calcification; this may occur in the presence of inadequate bone calcification due to the direct action of the vitamin on bone. Deposition of calcium in the kidneys leads to renal failure. It seems likely that idiopathic hypercalcaemia of infants is due to vitamin D overdosage.

1(d). *Abnormal vitamin D metabolism.* Hepatic metabolism of vitamin D is enhanced by antiepileptic therapy leading to a relative deficiency which may be overcome by dietary supplements. There is an inherited disorder in which renal 1α-hydroxylase is absent (autosomal recessive). Thus the most active renal metabolites of vitamin D cannot be produced. Massive dietary supplements normally overcome the problem. This is classical 'renal rickets'.

This condition must be distinguished from the sex-linked phosphaturic rickets in which there is a tubular anomaly reducing renal phosphate resorption.

1(*e*). *Hyperparathyroidism.* Isolated hyperparathyroidism is commonly due to an adenoma of one of the glands, but may be due to carcinoma.

The excessive secretion, by its direct action and by its effect upon vitamin D metabolism, causes raised serum calcium with a normal or low phosphate due to phosphaturia. Due to increased bone turnover the serum alkaline phosphatase is raised.

Symptoms include those due to hypercalcaemia including weakness, polyuria, gut problems, including peptic ulceration and renal stones. Generalized loss of bone occurs due to increased osteoclasis and at some sites may be so marked as to produce 'brown tumours'—giant-cell lesions with complete loss of bone. Such lesions are histologically indistinguishable from the giant-cell granuloma of the jaws. Brown tumours are not uncommon in the facial bones so it is important to distinguish between these two lesions, which means in practice excluding hyperparathyroidism by repeated examination of the serum calcium (*see* Chapter 10.

1(*f*). *Hypoparathyroidism.* This commonly results from thyroidectomy but may occur in the syndromes of hypoparathyroidism/hypoadrenalism/mucocutaneous candidosis and di George's syndrome (*see* Chapter 4).

Hypocalcaemia leads to increased neuromuscular excitability with tetany and epilepsy. Cataract formation is common.

Pseudohypoparathyroidism is an inherited disorder in which parathormone secretion is normal but there is renal hyporesponsiveness to the hormone. Patients suffer from mental retardation, tetany, epilepsy and extraosseous calcification.

1(*g*). *Uraemia.* In parenchymatous renal disease there is a progressive reduction in excretion of calcium and phosphate along with other ions. There is thus a tendency to hypercalcaemia and hyperphosphataemia. Due, however, to the diminished renal production of active metabolites of vitamin D, calcium absorption from the gut is reduced. The net effect being hyperphosphataemia. This leads to a tendency to hypocalcaemia probably by enhancing calcium deposition in bone. The hypocalcaemia stimulates hyperparathyroidism but the parathormone cannot exert its full effect on the renal tubules; inhibited from enhanced phosphate resorption by hyperphosphataemia and, as noted above, unable to stimulate the active metabolites of vitamin D in the kidney.

In addition, there is usually a well marked acidosis. This has the effect of substantially reducing ionized phosphate in spite of hyperphosphataemia.

Bone disease in early renal failure is osteomalacia with an element of hyperparathyroidism. As the disease progresses the parathyroid response becomes stronger and stronger, so that in advanced cases secondary hyperparathyroidism predominates.

The bone response may be modified by acidosis and other unidentified factors.

Clinically, bone disease is prominent in renal failure. Skeletal destruction from osteomalacia and hypoparathyroidism is marked. Extraskeletal calcification may also be prominent.

2(a). *Steroid hormones.* All the steroid hormones derived from the adrenal cortex and gonads have an influence on bone matrix production. Glucocorticoids promote catabolism of protein with generalized reduction in bone mass. Skeletal failure is one of the principal complications of long term steroid therapy and osteoporosis occurs in hyperadrenocorticism.

Diminished gonadal secretion also produces osteoporosis with reduced bone mass since these steroids are anabolic (they have the opposite effect upon bone from glucocorticoids).

In addition the onset of gonadal steroid production at puberty causes the epiphyses to close, so limiting height and limb length.

Corticosteroids tend to lower serum calcium, possibly by dimishing gut absorption. However calcium excretion is also enhanced. Bone turnover is reduced.

2(b) *Pituitary hormones (growth hormone).* In gigantism excess growth hormone enhances skeletal growth. Acromegaly produces enlargement of the acral (end) parts, including hands, feet, supraorbital ridges and mandible. Symmetrical enlargement of the mandible with prognathism and sometimes with spacing of the teeth is typical.

Surgery to reduce mandibular size in acromegaly should not be undertaken until the disease is controlled and even then is very hazardous due to the myopathy and cardiomyopathy of acromegaly, so is generally not indicated.

2(*b*). *Senile osteoporosis.* This is a generalized reduction in skeletal mass which generally produces symptoms in postmenopausal women. It occurs, but is generally less severe, in men.

The external size of 'anatomical' bones affected by osteoporosis is normal or increased but the volume of contained bone *tissue* is diminished, initially by reduction in the number of trabeculae in the spongiosa but later by thinning of cortical bone as well. The progressive loss of tissue seems to occur from about 40 years onward at about 10 per cent per annum, until the 7th decade when it stabilizes. The maximum bone density occurs on average in the 3rd decade.

The loss of bone mass is greater in postmenopausal women. As a result the bones become liable to fracture since they are less strong.

Although bone mass is reduced, and thus total body calcium, a negative calcium balance cannot be demonstrated. The serum calcium phosphate and alkaline phosphatase are normal. It is probably due (in part) to diminished gonadal steroid production and reduced stress on bone.

In a proportion of old people nutritional vitamin D deficiency or reduced metabolism or increased resistance to the action of the vitamin mean that borderline osteomalacia complicates the porosis. Up to 30 per cent of elderly patients suffering from fractures have histological evidence of osteomalacia.

There is no doubt that the elderly are subject to an increased incidence of fractures at 3 main sites—the vertebral bodies, the lower end of the radius and ulna (Colles fracture) and the neck of the femur.

2(*c*). *Thyroid.* Hyperthyroidism may be associated with osteoporosis and hypercalcaemia may occur. Thyroid hormone can apparently cause bone destruction and the resulting hypercalcaemia causes hyperparathyroidism.

3(*a*). *Generalized malignant disease* in bone is usually due to multiple metastases (carcinomatosis) or multifocal intraosseous neoplasia such as myelomatosis. Bone solution may be marked enough to produce symptoms of hypercalcaemia (vomiting), weakness and polyuria. In addition there may be bone pain, fractures and, on X-ray, multiple radiolucencies. The clinical picture may closely resemble hyperparathyroidism.

4(*a*). *Paget's disease of bone* is first noted in the 5th decade (1 per cent of men and 0·01 per cent of women) and the incidence rises progressively to about 8 per cent in men and 4 per cent in women in the 9th decade in post-mortem cases. Others have found a much higher incidence in radiological surveys (70 per cent in men and 30 per cent in women in the 7th decade).

The aetiology is unknown but there is a genetic tendency to the disease.

There is no apparent disturbance in calcium metabolism but serum alkaline phosphatase is always considerably raised.

The disease attacks individual bones in an apparently random fashion. One or many may be involved at one time or sequentially affecting particularly the pelvis, vertebrae and skull.

The involved bone becomes the seat of enhanced turnover with initially much destruction, softening and new bone formation. Eventually the bone becomes more dense and vascular than normal and remains enlarged (and possibly deformed).

If the jaws are affected the maxillae are usually involved; only rarely the mandible. Teeth in the affected jaw normally become extremely bulbous due to hypercementosis.

Calcitonin appears to be quite effective in treatment.

Pagetic bone is liable to an increased incidence of osteosarcomata of an unusually malignant form.

Appendix

A list of the more unusual syndromes which may affect the oral mucosa, with an outline of their principal features.

Acrodermatitis enteropathica (Danbolt–Closs syndrome)

Genetically determined abnormality of zinc metabolism.

Onset—between 9 months and 3 years, usually fatal but may improve after puberty.

Features—Mental disturbance, skin rash (perioral, perianal, hands and feet), oral and intestinal candidosis, diarrhoea, alopecia. Treated with zinc or di-iodohydroxyquin.

Acrodynia

Mercury intoxication, usually due to teething or worming powders.

Onset—between 9 months and 2 years.

Features—Extreme irritability, inflammation and desquamation of the skin of the hands, feet and face, sweating, salivation, tooth grinding (teeth may be exfoliated), oral ulceration, photophobia.

Ascher's syndrome

Hereditary disorder with a 'double' upper lip (an extreme laxity of the mucosal element of the lip), ptosis and non-toxic goitre.

Dyskeratosis congenita (Zinsser–Engman–Cole syndrome)

Genetically determined.

Features—At puberty the skin develops reticulated pigmentation with white atrophic areas. Tongue depapillated and recurrent oral bullae are seen. Progressive thickening of (white) plaques in the tongue occur. Histologically, they are dyskeratotic and carcinoma may supervene. The nails are dystrophic.

Fabry's syndrome (Angiokeratoma corporis diffusum universale)

Genetically determined (X-linked), deficiency of ceramide trihexosidase.

Features—Widespread telangiectatic lesions with overlying keratosis; occur on the skin, including lips, but *very rarely* oral mucosa. Severe intermittent acroparaesthesiae, also corneal opacities and progressive renal failure.

Focal dermal hypoplasia (Goltz' syndrome)

Features—Due to lobes in the *dermis* producing soft lobulation, fat herniated swellings with frail epidermal covering. Oral mucosal papillomatosis develops, also syndactyly, mental retardation, and hypodontia.

Gingival fibromatosis

This may be associated with mental retardation. Hypertrichosis.

Gustatary lacrimation

Lacrimation when eating which follows aberrant regrowth of parasympathetic fibres after facial palsy which extends proximal to the geniculate ganglion. (Not to be confused with Frey's syndrome of gustatary sweating due to aberrant regrowth of postganglionic fibres after severing the auriculotemporal nerve.)

Hyalinosis cutis et mucosae (lipoid proteinosis)

Features—Progressive waxy plaques in skin and mucosae; the oral mucosa is often most extensively involved. Tongue becomes progressively immobilized.

Incontinentia pigmentii (Bloch–Subzberger syndrome)

Genetically determined.

Features—Whorled cutaneous pigmentation with bullae. The teeth may be hypoplastic (conical) some may be supressed (hypodontia), but paradoxically supernumerary teeth also occur.

Lesch–Nyhan syndrome

Genetically determined deficiency of hypoxanthine-guanine phosphoribosyl transferase and consequent hyperuricaemia.

Features—Mental retardation, cerebral palsy and athetoid movements with self-mutilation (especially of the lips).

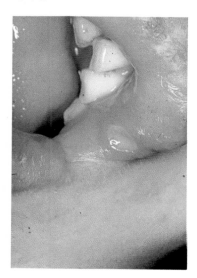

1
Aphthous ulcers

2
Aphthous ulcer
(major type)

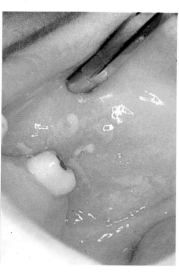

3
'Herpetiform'
aphthous ulcers

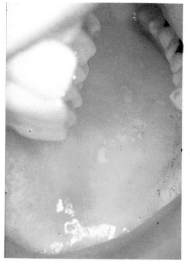

4
Pemphigus

5
Lichen planus
of the cheek

6
Erosive
lichen planus

7
Lichen planus
of the tongue

8
Geographical
tongue—
erythema
migrans linguae

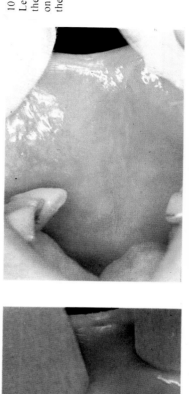

10 Leucoedema— the appearance on stretching the neck

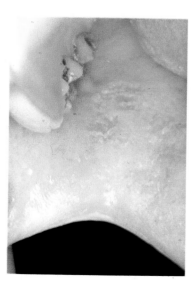

12 Black hairy tongue

9 Leucoedema—a typical 'fish-scale' appearance

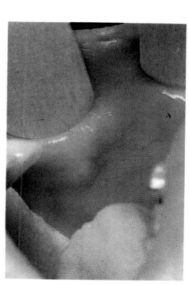

11 White sponge naevus of the cheek

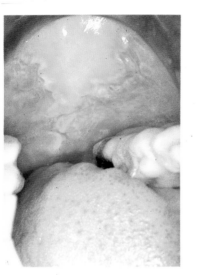

13
Chronic discoid
lupus
erythematosus

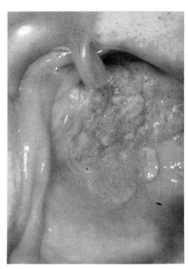

14
A further case
of lupus
erythematosus

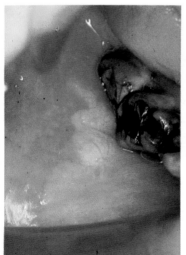

15
Squamous-cell
carcinoma of
the tongue

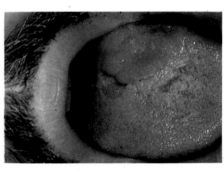

16
Extensive
'verrucous'
squamous-cell
carcinoma of
the palate

17
Xerostomia in
the sicca
syndrome

18
Carcinoma-
in-situ

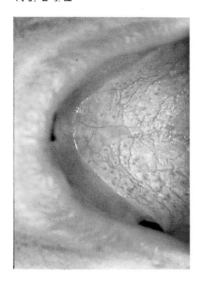

19
Chronic atrophic
candidosis of
the denture-
bearing area

20
Stomatitis
nicotinia—
smoker's
keratosis

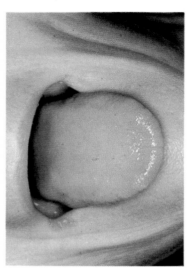

21
The pale
atrophic tongue
in iron-
deficiency
anaemia

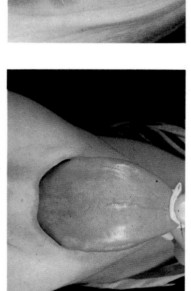

23
The inflamed
atrophic tongue
in pernicious
anaemia

22
Angular cheilitis
(candidal) in a
patient with
mild iron-
deficiency
anaemia

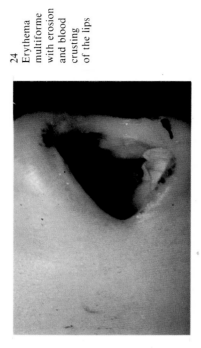

24
Erythema
multiforme
with erosion
and blood
crusting
of the lips

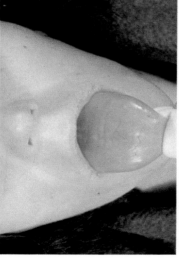

25
Idiopathic
pigmentation
of the mouth
resembling
the racial
pigmentation of
coloured peoples

26
Oral and
perioral
pigmentation
of the
Peutz – Jeghers
syndrome

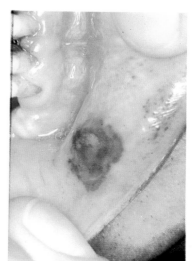

27
Oral
pigmentation in
Addison's
disease
(hypo-
adrenalism)

28
Bruising and
petechiae in
idiopathic
thrombo-
cytopaenic
purpura

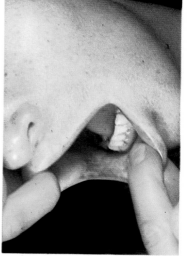

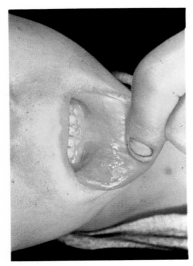

30
A mucous patch of secondary syphilis

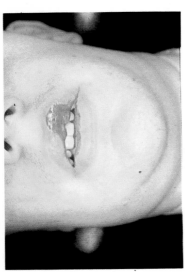

29
A primary chancre of the upper lip. Note the submandibular lymph-adenopathy

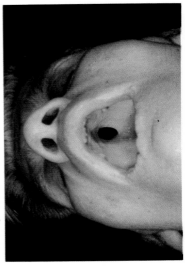

31
Gummatous perforation of the palate in tertiary syphilis

Index